New Techniques in the Psychotherapy of Older Patients

New Techniques in the Psychotherapy of Older Patients

Edited by

Wayne A. Myers, M.D.

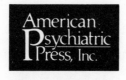

Washington, DC
London, England

Copyright © 1991 American Psychiatric Press, Inc.

ALL RIGHTS RESERVED

Manufactured in the United States of America on acid-free paper.

94 93 92 91   4   3   2   1
First Edition

American Psychiatric Press, Inc.
1400 K Street, N.W., Washington, DC 20005

Library of Congress Cataloging-in-Publication Data

New techniques in the psychotherapy of older patients / edited by Wayne A.
   Myers. — 1st ed.
     p.   cm.
   Includes bibliographical references.
   ISBN 0-88048-352-0 (alk. paper)
   1. Psychotherapy for the aged. I. Myers, Wayne A.
   [DNLM: 1. Psychotherapy—in old age. 2. Psychotherapy—
   methods. WT 150 N532]
   RC480.54.N49   1991
   618.97'68914—dc20
   DNLM/DLC
   for Library of Congress   90-14490
                                             CIP

British Library Cataloguing in Publication Data

A CIP record is available from the British Library.

Chap 1, 6, 14

CONTENTS

CONTRIBUTORS

Morton D. Bogdonoff, M.D.
Professor of Medicine
Cornell University Medical Center
New York, New York

Harry Bryan, M.D., Ed.D.
Staff Psychiatrist
Older Adult and Family Research and Resource Center
Division of Gerontology
Stanford University School of Medicine and
Palo Alto Veterans Administration Medical Center

Wayne Caron, M.A.
Project Coordinator
Alzheimer's Disease Clinical Research Center
Veterans Administration Medical Center
Minneapolis, Minnesota

Carl I. Cohen, M.D.
Professor of Psychiatry
Director of Geriatric Psychiatry
SUNY Health Science Center at Brooklyn, New York

Calvin A. Colarusso, M.D.
Clinical Professor of Psychiatry
University of California, San Diego
Training and Supervising Analyst
San Diego Psychoanalytic Institute

W. Edward Craighead, Ph.D.
Professor, Department of Psychiatry
Duke University Medical Center

John T. Curtis, Ph.D.
Co-Director, Brief Psychotherapy Research Project
Mt. Zion Hospital and Medical Center
Assistant Clinical Professor, Department of Psychiatry
University of California, San Francisco, Medical Center

Susan DelMaestro, Ph.D.
Staff Psychologist
Ambulatory Care Program
Philadelphia Veterans Administration Medical Center
Philadelphia, Pennsylvania

Sanford I. Finkel, M.D.
Director, Gero-Psychiatric Services
Northwestern Memorial Hospital
Associate Director, McGaw Center on Aging
Northwestern University

Margaret Florsheim, Ph.D.
Research Psychologist
Older Adult and Family Research and Resource Center
Division of Gerontology
Stanford University School of Medicine and
Palo Alto Veterans Administration Medical Center

Dolores Gallagher-Thompson, Ph.D.
Visiting Associate Professor
Counseling Psychology Program
Stanford University School of Education
Co-Director
Older Adult and Family Research and Resource Center

Frank Gantz, Psy.D.
Research Psychologist
Older Adult and Family Research and Resource Center
Division of Gerontology
Stanford University School of Medicine and
Palo Alto Veterans Administration Medical Center

Kenneth Hepburn, Ph.D.
Assistant Professor
Department of Family Practice and Community Health
University of Minnesota Medical School—Minneapolis

Jonathan Holt, M.D.
Assistant Professor of Psychiatry
Coordinator of Out-Patient Psychotherapy
Department of Psychiatry and Behavioral Sciences
SUNY at Stony Brook, New York

Teh-wei Hu, Ph.D.
Professor of Health Economics
University of California, Berkeley

D. Lynne Kaltreider, M.Ed.
Research Associate
Institute for Policy Research and Evaluation
The Pennsylvania State University

Helen Singer Kaplan, M.D., Ph.D.
Clinical Professor of Psychiatry
Director of Human Sexuality Program
New York Hospital–Cornell University Medical Center

Steven Lovett, Ph.D.
Lecturer, Division of Gerontology
Stanford University School of Medicine
Program Director, Division of Vision and Aging
Geriatric Research, Education and Clinical Center
Palo Alto Veterans Administration Medical Center

John R. Mach, Jr., M.D.
Medical Director
Geriatric Research, Education and Clinical Center
Veterans Administration Medical Center
Minneapolis, Minnesota
Instructor, Department of Medicine
University of Minnesota Medical School—Minneapolis

Mary Jane Massie, M.D.
Associate Professor of Clinical Psychiatry
New York Hospital–Cornell University Medical Center
Associate Attending Psychiatrist
Memorial–Sloan Kettering Hospital

Hindi T. Mermelstein, M.D.
Clinical Fellow at Memorial–Sloan Kettering Hospital
Fellow in Psychiatry
New York Hospital–Cornell University Medical Center

Patricia A. Miller, Ed.M., O.T.R.
Assistant Professor of Clinical Occupational Therapy and
  Public Health
Consultant, Center for Geriatrics and Gerontology
Columbia University

Wayne A. Myers, M.D.
Clinical Professor of Psychiatry
New York Hospital–Cornell University Medical Center
Training, Supervising and Admitting Psychoanalyst
Columbia University Center for Psychoanalytic Training and
Research

Robert A. Nemiroff, M.D.
Clinical Professor of Psychiatry
Director, Psychiatric Residency Training Program
Department of Psychiatry
University of California, San Diego
Training and Supervising Analyst
San Diego Psychoanalytic Institute

Jeffrey N. Nichols, M.D.
Clinical Assistant Professor of Medicine (Geriatrics and
  Gerontology)
New York Hospital–Cornell University Medical Center
Medical Director, Frances Schervier Home and Hospital
Bronx, New York

Jamie S. Ostroff, Ph.D.
Research Fellow, Memorial–Sloan Kettering Hospital
Fellow of Psychology in Psychiatry
New York Hospital–Cornell University Medical Center

John Rodman, Ph.D.
Research Psychologist
Older Adult and Family Research and Resource Center
Division of Gerontology
Stanford University School of Medicine and
Palo Alto Veterans Administration Medical Center

Steven P. Roose, M.D.
Associate Professor of Clinical Psychiatry
Columbia University College of Physicians and Surgeons
Research Psychiatrist, New York State Psychiatric Institute

Jon Rose, Ph.D.
Research Psychologist
Older Adult and Family Research and Resource Center
Division of Gerontology
Stanford University School of Medicine
Palo Alto Veterans Administration Medical Center

George Silberschatz, Ph.D.
Co-Director, Brief Psychotherapy Research Project
Mount Zion Hospital and Medical Center
Assistant Clinical Professor, Department of Psychiatry
University of California, San Francisco, Medical Center

Larry W. Thompson, Ph.D.
Professor of Medicine (Research)
Stanford University School of Medicine
Co-Director
Older Adult and Family Research and Resource Center

John A. Toner, Ed.D.
Assistant Professor of Clinical Public Health and Psychiatry
School of Public Health
Division of Geriatrics and Gerontology
Co-Director, New York State Geriatric Psychiatry Fellowship
Program, Center for Geriatrics and Gerontology
Columbia University Faculty of Medicine

Cheryl A. Walters, M.D.
Assistant Professor of Medicine
Cornell University Medical Center
Assistant Attending Physician
The New York Hospital
Director, Geriatrics Consultation Service

Lucy C. Yu, Ph.D.
Associate Professor of Health Policy and
Administration, College of Health and Human Development
The Pennsylvania State University

INTRODUCTION

In the past few decades, psychotherapy has undergone revolutionary changes. Not only are new techniques and medications available, but new populations have emerged that demand to be treated. Among the most important and rapidly growing of these new groups are the elderly. Whether we define them as the one-quarter of the U.S. populace over the age of 50 or the one-eighth of the country over the age of 65, this segment is already clamoring for greater attention and will do so increasingly in the next few decades.

Although numerous recent volumes (Lazarus 1984; Myers 1984; Nemiroff and Colarusso 1985; Sadavoy and Leszcz 1987) have described some of the basic psychotherapeutic techniques used with older patients, none has attempted to acquaint the reader with the truly remarkable variety of methods now being used in different parts of the country. *New Techniques in the Psychotherapy of Older Patients* attempts to redress this gap by offering a clinical as well as a theoretical look at these advanced new treatments.

The volume itself is divided into three sections. In the first, a variety of time-limited therapies that are used with older outpatients are described. The second section deals with shorter- and longer-term techniques that are used in the geriatrician's and psychotherapist's offices, as well as in the general hospital, the nursing home, and the chronic mental hospital. The third and final section of the book describes new approaches and new patient populations with whom longer-term treatment methods such as group therapy, psychoanalytic psychotherapy, and psychoanalysis are currently being applied.

The first time-limited technique to be described is that of cognitive-behavioral therapy. The chapter by Larry Thompson and his co-workers at Stanford University and at the Older Adult and Family Research and Resource Center at the Palo Alto Veterans Administration Hospital offers an overview of the cognitive therapy model of Aaron Beck (see Beck et al. 1979) as it is applied to the affective disorders of the elderly. The authors explain in detail how they attempt to reverse negative cognitive sets through various techniques geared to the identification and alteration of dysfunctional belief schemas.

The next chapter includes a description of the sex therapy employed by Helen Singer Kaplan at the Payne Whitney Clinic of Cornell University Medical Center. Dr. Kaplan notes that for older persons to remain sexually functional, they must adapt to specific age-related changes in their sexual response. She describes these changes and offers a detailed case vignette of her work with a couple who is experiencing difficulties in adapting to the problems of their aging. The methods employed in her treatment program involve an amalgam of behavioral approaches to deal with the current causes of the sexual dysfunctions and the utilization of specific psychodynamic techniques to deal with the deeper emotional and marital difficulties. In addition, physical and laboratory examinations performed to rule out any underlying organic disorders that may be causing or complicating the presenting picture are outlined.

In the next chapter, Kenneth Hepburn and colleagues from the University of Minnesota Medical School—Minneapolis and the Minneapolis Veterans Administration Medical Center offer a family therapy approach to the problems of caregivers of patients afflicted with chronic illnesses or impairments. The authors note that about 80% of the in-home care needs of the chronically impaired elderly are met by families. Caregiving has a negative impact on the mental and physical health of the caregiver. Important manifestations in the caregivers are a markedly increased prevalence of depression and the overall sense of being burdened. Hepburn and his co-workers enumerate their principles of care geared toward helping to conserve the well-being of the family caregivers. They use a variety of methods in their work, including individual counseling with a brief problem-oriented focus, supportive therapy, and interventions intended to reduce stress. Family therapy per se is employed to make certain that the family serves as a resource to the caregiver and not as a further source of stress.

In a similar vein, Dolores Gallagher-Thompson, Steven Lovett, and Jon Rose from Stanford University and the Palo Alto Veterans Administration Medical Center also discuss the types of interventions utilized with stressed family caregivers. The authors detail their work with life satisfaction, problem solving, and anger-management classes. They also describe the effectiveness of two forms of brief psychotherapy—a cognitive-behavioral approach and Mann's (1973) time-limited psychodynamic psychotherapy—that they used in treating the acute psychopathology of caregivers through their work with Project Assist. A number of illustrative case examples are included to demonstrate the effectiveness of the particular methods employed and to indicate the importance of such time-limited methods in dealing with the profound problems besetting the ever-growing group of caregivers for the elderly.

Carl Cohen, the director of Geriatric Psychiatry at the SUNY Health Science Center in Brooklyn, New York, describes his community-based work employing social-network techniques with the marginal elderly (such as residents of single-room-occupancy hotels) in New York. He describes the use of the Network Analysis Profile, which enables him to investigate the quantitative and qualitative features of various social networks. Clinically, this approach uses the older person's social network to deal with his or her problems. Network sessions involving the families and friends of clients are used, as are individually centered treatment approaches. Case examples are included to show what sorts of interventions are made, and a description of which populations do best with such approaches is included.

As the final chapter in this section, George Silberschatz and John Curtis of the Mount Zion Hospital and Medical Center in San Francisco offer another variety of time-limited psychotherapy that they have employed with older patients. Their 16 weekly psychodynamically oriented psychotherapy sessions work on disconfirming pathogenic expectations of the patients vis-à-vis the therapists. According to their view, when the therapists pass certain "tests," the patients are likely to become more productively involved in the therapeutic work. They also find the concept of survivor guilt to be particularly useful in understanding older patients' resistance to treatment. The authors offer a variety of cogent clinical examples to advance their theoretical viewpoint.

The second section of the book begins with a sophisticated chapter on the diagnosis and pharmacological treatment of depression in older patients by Steven Roose of the Columbia University College of Physicians and Surgeons and the New York State Psychiatric Institute. This chapter is included to emphasize that no volume on psychotherapy of older patients would be meaningful if it arbitrarily separated psychotherapeutic techniques from pharmacotherapeutic ones. Most often it is only through the thorough knowledge and combination of both modalities that we can offer the best possible treatment program to our older patients. In Roose's chapter, after a thoughtful section on the prevalence of depression in the population over age 65, he spells out the criteria used in the differential diagnosis of depression. An informative discussion of the pharmacological treatment of this disorder follows. Important sections here include a detailed description of the pharmacokinetic factors influencing the dosage of medications such as the tricyclic antidepressants in elderly patients and a delineation of the concepts of adequate versus partial treatment of these disorders.

Because many elderly patients never reach the psychotherapist's office, but are treated instead by internists or geriatricians, the next chapter describes various therapeutic interventions offered to such individuals by a team of geriatricians at the Cornell University Medical Center. Nichols, Walters, and Bogdonoff first discuss the types of patients most frequently evaluated by the geriatrician: individuals with cognitive disorders, depressions, and other chronic psychiatric problems and those with somatic complaints. Evaluations involve ruling out a variety of medical conditions that may present with psychiatric symptoms and an examination of the types of medications being used,which also may induce or aggravate mental problems. Following this, Nichols offers a number of interesting case vignettes to illustrate the way in which they bounce back and forth between the use of medical regimens and psychotherapeutic techniques. The latter often include positive environmental manipulations and a multidisciplinary approach aimed at reducing the artificial polarization between mind and body in patients and their families.

From the geriatrician's office, we move on to the treatment of the elderly cancer patient in the chapter by Hindi Mermelstein, Jamie Ostroff, and Mary Jane Massie from the Psychiatry Service of the Memorial–Sloan-Kettering Hospital. As the authors note, individuals over age 65 account for one-half of the cancer cases in the United States. Psychological issues arise at various times in the treatment of such patients. Some are seen immediately after learning that they are suffering from cancer. Other problems arise during the universally stressful period of active cancer treatment. In this phase, various psychotherapeutic interventions are used, including supportive and behavioral approaches and pharmacological agents. Suicide is a problem that must be guarded against during this period. After active treatment, other psychological issues arise during the palliative and terminal phases of medical management and in the period of survivorhood. Clinical vignettes are presented to document the wide variety of multimodal interventions that the authors prescribe for their patients.

The next chapter, by Jonathan Holt from the Health Science Campus of SUNY at Stony Brook, deals with hypnotherapeutic interventions used with older patients. Holt details a variety of hypnotic techniques in a number of clinical case examples. The interplay between direct and indirect suggestions, other forms of psychotherapy, and the use of medication is quite elucidating.

Lucy Yu, D. Lynne Kaltreider, Teh-wei Hu, and W. Edward Craighead, from the Health Policy Section at The Pennsylvania State University, the Health Economics Section at the University of California, Berkeley, and the Department of Psychiatry of the Duke University Medical Center, describe the impact of a behavior therapy approach on the psychological status of incontinent elderly nursing home residents. The authors note that whereas only 9% of the elderly in the community experience incontinence, 40–50% of such individuals in nursing homes are incontinent. The economic costs of coping with this problem are staggering and account for at least 10% of the total nursing-home-care costs in our country. The authors studied 133 elderly women from seven Pennsylvania nursing homes in a randomized clinical trial to evaluate the effectiveness of prompted toileting on the participants' urinary incontinence. The data indicated that the behavior therapy program was effective in reducing the incidence of incontinence among the women in the treatment group. Although they were unable to statistically document significant changes in the psychosocial status of the participants in the program, members of the project team observed such changes in some of the women and felt that these findings have important implications for health care providers and policy makers.

The last chapter in this section describes the evolution of a geriatric team at the Willard Psychiatric Center in New York State, as part of a study under the auspices of the New York State Geriatric Psychiatry Fellowship Program and the Center for Geriatrics and Gerontology of Columbia University. The authors, Patricia Miller and John Toner of Columbia University, applied an interdisciplinary approach that had evolved over a number of years at the Willard Psychiatric Center. Team members volunteered to work in the experimental unit, which offered an innovative clinical program for the care of patients with dementia who were at risk for losing mobility. The team was encouraged to develop a manual and goals for themselves and to use problem-solving techniques to fulfill their goals. The authors describe, with appropriate clinical examples, their techniques in honing the requisite knowledge and skills for the team's development, management, and maintenance.

The final section of the book begins with a chapter by Sanford Finkel, past secretary of the International Psycho-Geriatric Society and director of Gero-Psychiatric Services at the Northwestern Memorial Hospital in Chicago, on the use of group therapy with older patients. Finkel points out the cost-effectiveness of treating patients in groups and notes that this technique can be used in inpatient and nursing home settings, as well as in dealing with outpatients. Among the special advantages of this type of treatment are the development of a sense of identity as part of a social entity and the feeling of nurture and support afforded by the group setting. Finkel outlines a number of important issues that arise in working with older groups, including the characteristics required of the group leader, the ideal number of patients for such a group, and the themes and goals of groups for this specific population. In addition, he details some of the similarities and differences between groups composed of older and of younger people.

In the next chapter, Calvin Colarusso and Robert Nemiroff, from the University of California, San Diego, present some of their ground-breaking work on the impact of adult developmental issues in the treatment of older persons. They initially note some of the important developmental tasks of late adulthood and, by use of cogent case examples, illustrate how this knowledge influences the choice of psychotherapeutic modality employed with patients in this age range. They advocate detailed diagnostic evaluations to collect relevant data and to differentiate between normal and deviant developments in their patients. The authors note some of the countertransference issues experienced by younger therapists working with older patients and also describe various specialized therapeutic techniques applicable to elderly patients.

In the final chapter, I present some of my own experiences in working with older patients in psychoanalytically oriented psychotherapy and in psychoanalysis. I describe some of the problems inherent in evaluating which patients will do best with either one or the other of these specific treatment modalities. A number of different factors are described that enter into such decisions. Clinical examples relevant to these specific factors are included. In addition, case material illustrating the different kinds of interventions made in the particular treatments are described to familiarize the reader with these techniques.

This volume attempts to present the state-of-the-art methods of psychotherapy available for use with older patients in the United States. Although we may have overemphasized certain varieties of treatment and underplayed others, we have tried to make the coverage fair and comprehensive. It is clear that this is an evolving field, and we will soon be seeing cognitive-behavioral and other time-limited methods of psychotherapy being employed in settings as diverse as sex therapy clinics, nursing homes, and chronic mental hospitals.

What we are seeing is a treatment revolution, and we must all be open to the panoply of techniques available to psychotherapists of all persuasions. Even though some of the older patients we treat may be senile, we must not allow our own thinking to become ossified. It is toward this openness of spirit that this book is dedicated.

REFERENCES

Beck AT, Rush AJ, Shaw BF, et al: Cognitive Therapy of Depression. New York, Guilford, 1979

Lazarus LW (ed): Clinical Approaches to Psychotherapy With the Elderly. Washington, DC, American Psychiatric Press, 1984

Mann J: Time-Limited Psychotherapy. Cambridge, MA, Harvard University Press, 1973

Myers WA: Dynamic Therapy of the Older Patient. New York, Jason Aronson, 1984

Nemiroff RA, Colarusso CA (eds): The Race Against Time: Psychotherapy and Psychoanalysis in the Second Half of Life. New York, Plenum, 1985

Sadavoy J, Leszcz M (eds): Treating the Elderly With Psychotherapy: The Scope for Change in Later Life. Madison, CT, International Universities Press, 1987

BRIEF PSYCHOTHERAPEUTIC TREATMENTS

Chapter One

COGNITIVE-BEHAVIORAL THERAPY FOR AFFECTIVE DISORDERS IN THE ELDERLY

Larry W. Thompson, Ph.D., Frank Gantz, Psy.D.,
Margaret Florsheim, Ph.D., Susan DelMaestro, Ph.D.,
John Rodman, Ph.D., Dolores Gallagher-Thompson, Ph.D.,
and Harry Bryan, M.D., Ed.D.

In this chapter we hope to provide the reader with an introduction to the use of cognitive-behavioral (CB) psychotherapy in treating emotional distress in the elderly. We discuss a number of problems that often bring elderly individuals into treatment, briefly describe several frequently used CB intervention techniques, and present a case example illustrating the process of treatment. The chapter concludes with our observations about the characteristics of patients for whom this type of therapy generally works well versus those who do not seem to benefit as much. We also include some research data on the efficacy of this therapy modality, especially for late-life depression. The chapter assumes that the reader is familiar with the conceptual model and techniques used in CB therapy. Detailed information about specific concepts and intervention strategies can be found in Beck et al. (1979).

COMMON PROBLEMS THAT BRING OLDER PERSONS INTO THERAPY

Many of the normal changes associated with aging can be stressful and can result in emotional distress. Numerous developmental tasks of late adulthood, such as the need to cope with loss of significant

Considerable support for this project has been provided by the National Institute of Mental Health (Grants MH-37196 and MH-40041).

others and with changes in one's own physical well-being, can present unique therapeutic issues. Common presenting problems of older adults seeking psychotherapy fall into categories of life-style changes, bereavement, relationship problems, and health-related difficulties. These categories are somewhat arbitrary, and some presenting problems fall into several categories at once; however, these groupings were chosen because they represent areas of problematic adjustment for many older persons.

Life-Style Changes

Common life-style changes include retirement, relocation, and change in financial status. While many individuals face these events without distress, some older adults respond to these events by developing a clinical level of depression or anxiety. CB theorists conceptualize these responses as being directly related to an individual's perceptions of major life events. Many maladaptive belief systems may be triggered by life-style crises. For example, individuals who believe that their life is only meaningful as long as they are making money may respond to retirement with thoughts that they no longer have worth and are out of the mainstream of society. Consequently, they are more susceptible to feelings of depression. In addition, when life-style changes occur, many sources of positive reinforcement may disappear. Relocation, for instance, can result in loss of immediate contact with acquaintances and friends who have provided the individual with positive feedback and a sense of meaningfulness in the community.

Bereavement

Old age is typically accompanied by the deaths of spouse, family, and friends and, ultimately, the end of one's own life. Bereavement is thus an all-too-common experience in the years after age 60. Another form of loss is experienced by older adults who are caregivers for frail elders. The change in relationship that occurs when one party is cognitively or physically impaired and requires assistance can be experienced as a major loss of things that might have been. Facing the end of one's own life can lead to reflection on its meaning and quality. It can also mean facing missed opportunities, relationships that were never resolved, and life goals that were never achieved. Common thoughts that may arise in individuals feeling overwhelming distress when faced with loss of others may be "I can't survive alone," "He had no right to leave me," "My life is filled with failure,"

4

and "I will never again be as close to anyone as the friends I've lost." Loss of friends and family may also lead to a narrowing of a person's opportunities for social interaction and involvement in activities that are pleasurable and self-enhancing.

Relationship Problems

Marital issues and problems with children can occur throughout the life span. However, there are special circumstances associated with aging that can negatively impact long-standing, significant relationships. For example, a couple that maintained stability in their relationship by limiting time spent together and putting energy into work commitments may experience increased conflict and discomfort upon retirement. They may lack the skills needed to plan pleasant shared activities or communicate their needs for time alone. In addition, their beliefs about how relationships should be structured, which have developed over the history of the relationship, may now be incompatible with the changes resulting from retirement. For example, a woman who has served in the role of housewife may think, "The home is my territory. He's always interfering because he probably thinks I can't do anything right on my own." Other marital relationship problems can also occur when one or both of the partners become ill and the balance of their dependence on each other shifts. They may have to assume new responsibilities that make them more aware of skill deficits and result in feelings of inadequacy. Spouses' attributions about behavioral changes associated with illness as well as role adjustments in the marriage can result in negative affect. For example, a wife whose husband has suffered cognitive changes from a stroke may attribute her husband's altered behavior to laziness or lack of caring for her. She may think "He's doing this on purpose. He only cares about himself. If he really loved me, he'd do what I ask."

In addition, many older adults have relationship conflicts with their adult children. Some elderly persons still provide emotional and monetary support for their children and may become involved in unhelpful "codependent" relationships. The elder's role in creating many of these difficulties appears to be based on their continuing sense of responsibility for their adult children. This may be manifested in such beliefs as "I have to be there to rescue my alcoholic daughter or else her life and my grandchildren's lives will be ruined." Another form of relationship difficulty can occur when elders relocate to live closer to their children. This adjustment may result in emotional stress for all parties. Older adults who have placed primary emphasis on their relationship with their children may become disappointed when they cannot find a place in their children's hectic life-style. Others may find that their children have more expectations for contact than they want and may find it hard to develop an independent life-style in their new location.

Health-Related Difficulties

While good health may be maintained throughout much of one's lifetime, many older adults must adjust to chronic or acute illnesses. For example, an active elderly woman who breaks her hip or an older gentleman with arthritis who can no longer play golf regularly may become "homebound" and feel extremely isolated and depressed. The cognitive-behaviorist understands that this kind of emotional distress results from nonadaptive thoughts and behavioral responses to the health changes that have occurred. For example, typical thoughts might be, "If I can't be as active as I once was, my life has little meaning" and "No one wants to be around someone who is sick. I'm only a burden to them." These thoughts may result in unhelpful cognitive interpretations of health changes and make the individual more susceptible to feelings of depression, anxiety, and anger. Behaviorally, physical disability can result in decreased involvement in enjoyed activities and a sense of reduced satisfaction and pleasure in life. Additionally, elders facing physical limitations may find themselves having to rely on others for tasks they were once able to do on their own. Those who lack the skills necessary to communicate their special needs to others may feel distress when their needs are not met.

In summary, then, a variety of situations may occur that result in serious depression and/or anxiety for an older person. In our experience, the four kinds of situations detailed above are the most common and represent the kinds of changes and perceptions that are most amenable to CB therapy. After briefly outlining a number of common CB techniques in the next section, we will present a case example that illustrates the use of CB therapy with outpatients presenting with these kinds of problems.

SIMILARITIES AND DIFFERENCES IN CB THERAPY WITH OLDER AND YOUNGER ADULTS AND DESCRIPTIONS OF CURRENT TECHNIQUES

Therapy with older adults is very similar to that with younger persons in many respects. Like others, older clients enter treatment during various stages of the change process, with biases, expectations, and differing degrees of motivation to change. The content of presenting problems tends to differ, as mentioned above, but an elder's emotional and behavioral reactions are not so distinct as may be imagined. Even problems such as eating disorders, previously believed to be restricted to the young, can sometimes be found in older adults (Stelnick and Thompson 1989).

Nevertheless, while similarities far outweigh differences, certain modifications in the implementation of treatment seem to be necessary. The elderly are a more heterogeneous group than other age groups, and this fact requires flexibility in the therapist. Because of cohort effects (e.g., social and historical), there is greater variability in educational level, interests, current life situation, and physical and intellectual functioning (Troll 1985). Thus, the clinician should conduct a thorough psychological and social assessment, obtain a medical history, and confer with the patient's primary physician about current health status and medications in order to be sensitive to the many factors that may be operating in a given situation.

In addition to some differences in content of therapy, the process of CB therapy in the elderly may contrast with that used with younger patients. (See Thompson et al. [1986] and Emery [1981] for further discussion of this issue.) One major difference is that the therapist needs to be more active with an older client, keeping him or her focused and maintaining the structure of the session. There is sometimes a tendency for older clients, who are often lonely, to digress from the task at hand and engage in "storytelling." With a "captive audience," there is a temptation to share additional material not related to the therapeutic objectives. While some of this life review material may be clinically rich and relevant, the therapist must use his or her clinical judgment and typically redirect the patient's focus to the "here and now" problem that brought him or her into therapy.

Therapy with older persons generally proceeds at a slightly slower pace. One reason is that some elders suffer a loss of visual or auditory capacity. Significant hearing loss occurs in about 30% of the older population (Butler and Gastel 1979) and can affect the rate (not to mention the accuracy) at which auditory information is processed. Therapists should inquire about hearing loss and make the appropriate accommodations. The therapist will also do well to speak more slowly than usual and to enunciate clearly, since unclear speech can further interfere with comprehension.

Another important issue involves the possibility that elders may not learn at the same rate or in the same manner as younger persons and may be at a disadvantage in using inductive reasoning and ab-

7

stract verbal processing (Willis 1985). Depression and other negative affective states can influence cognitive processes and the learning of new information. One strategy for minimizing possible psychological obstructions with any client is, of course, the building of rapport and the promotion of a strong working alliance. Relationship variables are just as important in CB therapy as in any other approach and have begun to receive more attention in the behavioral literature (Kanfer and Grimm 1980). One way of building rapport is to adopt the older patient's own language when addressing important issues. This shows respect for his or her perceptions. Encouraging the client to "teach" the therapist something is also very helpful in that it reduces the status difference between the client and therapist. The subject can be as mundane as the "short-cut" used to get to the office. In addition, analogies used in the course of treatment might be framed in terms of the client's primary lifetime occupation, making them more meaningful (Pankrantz and Kofoed 1988).

In terms of grappling with cognitive slowing or sensory deficits, it is helpful to present important information in several different sensory modalities. For example, one might repeat important themes or concepts both verbally and visually (e.g., using a blackboard) as well as have the patient take notes. One might also provide a tape recording of the interview for review between sessions, particularly for those patients exhibiting more severe sensory and/or cognitive impairment. Handouts and written feedback can also facilitate the integration of important therapeutic concepts and material. Asking the client to reiterate major themes at the end of the session can also help some patients to encode and integrate at a deeper cognitive level what is learned in treatment.

Socialization to Treatment

In CB therapy, a collaborative relationship is considered essential. Such a relationship may radically differ from the older person's expectations regarding the nature of therapy, particularly if the patient has had other forms of treatment. Therefore, care must be taken in setting up the therapeutic relationship because the patient may misinterpret a collaborative stance as a sign of the therapist's lack of confidence. The CB approach is usually presented as an active learning process requiring the full participation of the client. Ideally, an atmosphere of "collaborative empiricism" is created in which the patient's dysfunctional attitudes and behaviors are framed as hypotheses to be tested.

Another key issue in the socialization process is homework. Elders

8

usually are far removed from the educational model and "homework" may be perceived as "childish" or unnecessary. However, homework plays an integral role in treatment because applying what is learned in therapy is critical to fostering a transfer of skills to the patient's home environment and speeds patient progress (Beck and Emery 1985; Gallagher and Thompson 1983).

Regardless of the patient's prior therapy experience, the therapist should solicit the patient's general expectations of therapy and stereotypes about the process of change. This issue is particularly salient in the treatment of older adults because this cohort may have strong negative beliefs about what it means to be in therapy (e.g., "Therapy is for crazy people") (Emery 1981). Another common cognitive obstacle to treatment is the belief that "I am too old to change." One way to intervene is to reframe the goal of therapy, emphasizing the learning of new coping skills. Implicit in all of this, of course, is that the clinician is aware of his or her own beliefs and expectations with regard to working with older adults.

In addition to specific problematic beliefs such as those above, patients may display deeply ingrained problem-solving approaches to which they rigidly adhere. The therapist may have to be creative in engaging the patient to explore alternative problem-solving approaches. One way of intervening is to frame the new approach as a temporary experiment in which data will be gathered to evaluate the approach's effectiveness.

COMMON AND EFFECTIVE CB TECHNIQUES

In the 9 years that our center has been in operation, we have utilized a variety of cognitive and behavioral techniques with older adults, reflecting the large number of techniques in the CB armamentarium. However, this section will focus on those we have found to be particularly helpful and/or have modified for use with elders (see Table 1-1). For the interested reader, excellent compendiums of cognitive techniques can be found in Burns (1980, 1989) or McMullin (1986). Goldfried and Davison (1976) provide a thorough overview of clinical behavior therapy and Lewinsohn et al. (1986) also provide a useful reference. For books dealing specifically with the treatment of elders, see Gallagher and Thompson (1981) or Hussian and Davis (1985).

Cognitive Techniques

Dysfunctional thought records. The most frequently used cognitive technique is the Dysfunctional Thought Record (DTR) (see Table 1-

Table 1-1. Cognitive and behavioral techniques particularly useful with elders

---

Cognitive
  Dysfunctional Thought Record (DTR)
  Generating alternative thoughts
  Vertical arrow technique
  Evaluating the evidence

Behavioral
  Daily mood monitoring
  Older Person's Pleasant Events Schedule
  Journal writing (activities, events, or thoughts)
  Assertiveness training
  Relaxation training

---

2). Initially, the DTR can be used to illustrate the relationship between thoughts and emotions. Later, it can be used directly to identify and challenge the dysfunctional thoughts related to the patient's negative emotional states. At our center, we have developed several simplified formats geared to match the patient's needs and level of understanding. For example, some patients find the generation of adaptive thoughts to be quite difficult at first. One simplified format addressing this issue includes a space for writing out not only the automatic thought, but also the cognitive distortion that the thought represents, and then space for writing out an adaptive response to the distortion. Identification of the specific cognitive distortion (see Table 1-3) facilitates the process of learning to challenge automatic thoughts by giving the patient a point of entry into his or her maladaptive thinking. Meanwhile, the challenging of thoughts is devel-

Table 1-2. Partially completed Dysfunctional Thought Record

Situation	Emotion and extent	Dysfunctional thoughts
Waiting for my son to call; it is Sunday evening, late, and he has not yet called even though I had expected him to do so by now.	Depression 70% Anger 80%	Something must have happened to him. No, more likely I have said or done something to offend him. Why does this always happen to me, that I am disappointed and people let me down?

Table 1-3. Partial listing of convenient cognitive distortions

1. *All-or-nothing thinking*: Seeing things in terms of black and white, with no gray areas.
2. *Mental filter*: Selectively attending to certain classes of events; "negative scanning."
3. *Jumping to conclusions*: Includes "mindreading," or acting as if one knows what others are thinking, and "fortune telling," or predicting future calamities.
4. *Emotional reasoning*: Believing something is true because you feel it is so ("I feel like a failure, so I must be one").
5. *Should and implied should statements*: Making opinions into absolute rules using words like "should," "must," and "ought," or beliefs that imply such a process.

Source. Adapted from Burns 1980, pp. 40–41.

oped in therapy, and another DTR format can be substituted when the patient has developed some proficiency in disputation.

In practice, the therapist is usually presented with a negative emotion connected to a particular situation, such as "I'm angry and hurt because my son didn't call me on Sunday." This is placed in the "situation" column (Table 1-2). The level of depression, anxiety, or anger can then be rated, e.g., 80%, and placed in the "emotions" column. The therapist then can begin to probe the client's thinking by asking questions like "What went through your mind when you didn't hear from him? What did you tell yourself about that? or What did you say to yourself to get upset about him not calling you?" The client may respond "Well, he never calls me! He doesn't care about me at all!" These thoughts are placed in the "dysfunctional thoughts" column and we approach the quintessence of cognitive therapy. Based on the above, the following case material illustrates several techniques used in changing automatic thoughts.

Identifying Cognitive Distortions

Therapist: Now that we've got it all on the DTR, let's look at what you told yourself. Do you see any distortions in your thinking, like the ones we discussed last week?

Client: Well, I said "never." That's not really true.

T: Overgeneralization, maybe?

C: Yes, I suppose.

T: And what about the "he doesn't care" part? How do you know that is true?

C: Well, I guess I don't. I'm "mindreading" again.

Generating Alternative Thoughts

T: Are those helpful thoughts to have? Could you have said something different to yourself?

C: No, they upset me. I could have said, "Just because he didn't call doesn't mean he doesn't care. He may be busy today. He does have that big project at work."

T: Okay, and what happens to your anger when you think that?

C: Well, it's true, I do feel less angry, only about 50%. But it seems like he never calls me!

Evaluating the Evidence

T: Okay, well, we're not finished. You've said that this could be over-generalization, but it sounds like it's hard for you to believe it. Let's examine the evidence for your thought that he "never" calls. When was the last time he called?

C: Don't know. Been so long I can't remember.

T: Think a moment. (Pause)

C: Well, he called last week to see how I was doing. That was Thursday, from work. And he called last Sunday, too. I guess he calls, but he doesn't like to talk very long. He doesn't like the phone. I still feel angry and hurt.

Vertical Arrow Technique

T: It seems like there is more to this. You can't seem to let go of the hurt and anger. What does it mean about you if your son doesn't talk to you or call you enough? What does it mean about you as a person?

C: About me? Well, it must mean he doesn't love me.

T: Uh-huh. And if he doesn't love you, then what?

C: Well, if he doesn't love me, I've done something wrong. But that's personalizing, isn't it?

T: That's correct, but let's not work on distortions right now. What do you believe about yourself if he doesn't love you?

C: If he doesn't love me . . . if he doesn't love me, his own mother, then I must be a terrible person. I am a complete failure!

T: It sounds like you believe that if you don't have your son's complete love, you are nothing in life, a complete failure. This seems to be a deeper belief you have. Perhaps that has something to do with why you moved closer to him. This thought is one we'll have to work on for awhile, until you can believe that your self-worth has nothing to do with your son's love for you.

The "vertical arrow" works backward along the client's chain of reasoning until arriving at his or her erroneous premise, in this case that a mother's worth is measured by how much love and attention she receives from her child. The cognitive therapist would continue to work with this "core belief" focusing on the evidence for and against this belief, looking for inevitable variations on the theme. Frequently, deeper assumptions or beliefs such as these form overarching cognitive structures that can result in thematic patterns of automatic thoughts for clients. However, not all thoughts need to be related in this way, and the identification of a core belief is not necessary for cognitive therapy to be productive.

Behavioral Techniques

With more depressed patients, it is often essential to begin therapy using behavioral interventions. The cognitive model can appear overwhelming to a depressed client because it is more complex. Behavioral assignments and rationale are easier for the client to understand, help to break through the depressive inertia, increase mood, and, if successfully applied, create positive expectations for the rest of therapy.

Daily mood monitoring is often one of the first interventions utilized. Clients track their mood between sessions, rate the level of depression, and give one or two reasons why they think they felt the way they did or mention daily events. This is particularly useful for psychologically naive persons who are unable to identify why they feel the way they do. Not only does this help identify stressors, but the practice highlights mood variability over the course of several weeks, which can often be a surprise to clients. Used in conjunction with the Pleasant Events Schedule (see below), this can be a powerful intervention.

A behavioral concomitant of depression that serves to exacerbate the condition is a reduction in pleasant activities (Lewinsohn et al. 1986). The Older Person's Pleasant Events Schedule (Gallagher and Thompson 1981) has become one of the more frequently used interventions at our center. Measures of both the frequency of pleasant events and the subjective pleasure derived from them are evaluated in this questionnaire, providing an objective picture of the patient's pleasant activities over the preceding month. From this information, interventions that focus on increasing the frequency of pleasant events can be developed. Alternatively, cognitive techniques can be used to increase the perception of pleasure when anhedonia exists. The measure can also be used to assess change at different points in therapy. A partial listing of items from this schedule is presented in Table 1-4.

Another rather flexible technique found to be highly useful is journal writing (self-monitoring). Frequently, depressed elders will under- or overestimate the frequency of certain events (e.g., they are "not getting any housework done"). Keeping a journal not only pro-

Table 1-4. Sample items from the Older Person's Pleasant Events
Schedule

Having coffee, tea, etc., with friends.
Listening to the sounds of nature.
Being told I am needed.
Giving advice to others based on past experience.
Visiting a museum.
Feeling a sense of accomplishment.
Having positive memories.

Note. Items are rated separately for frequency on a 3-point scale from did not occur to occurred several times a week, and pleasantness on a similar 3-point scale from not pleasant to very pleasant or enjoyable, so that the therapist can select particular items with a discrepancy, i.e., those that are done infrequently but would give pleasure if they occurred.

vides the clinician with better data, but, more important, also can be quite therapeutic for the patient.

Lack of assertiveness skills is a common problem for many psychotherapy clients and elders are no exception. When working with elders in this regard, treat with empathy fears of rejection by the patient's significant others, which may inhibit more adaptive behavior. Older persons are very aware of the possibility of becoming more dependent on family members and may fear retaliation in the future, sometimes with good reason. An empathic approach emphasizing graduated escalations of assertive behavior, as well as the gathering of outcome data, is extremely helpful in assuring an appropriate and safe intervention.

Finally, use of any of a number of standard methods of relaxation training helps clients to gain a sense of mastery over anxiety, which in turn facilitates therapeutic progress in general.

The following vignette (identifying data have been thoroughly obscured) illustrates the use of various CB strategies with older men and women experiencing different kinds of affective disorders and responses to common changes associated with aging. At our center, we routinely conduct 3-, 6-, and 12-month posttherapy follow-up evaluation interviews with our patients, so information available from the follow-up is included whenever possible.

Mr. D. is a 76-year-old widowed man who came to our center initially complaining of feelings of depression. At intake, he reported having mild arthritis, arteriosclerosis, and hypertension. His physician had prescribed trazodone for depression, an antihypertensive, and an anticoagulant.

The process of therapy was characterized by a high level of compliance and very real therapeutic gains in spite of the significant health problems. Mr. D.'s treatment progressed rapidly due to previous experience with CB therapy, his level of motivation, and, unfortunately, a desire to please the therapist and to "look good." (This last factor emerged late in the course of treatment, as will be seen.) An independent evaluation prior to treatment yielded a diagnosis of major depressive disorder.

Mr. D.'s initial complaint was of "not doing anything at home." This was assessed for one week using a journal of daily activities. At the second session, the patient was very surprised and pleased to see that, indeed, he was quite active and productive. Thus, the assessment procedure had immediate therapeutic value (often the case with this technique). Actually, the main problem was that Mr. D. had minimized both the amount and importance of his work, including the handiwork he had done regularly for his granddaughter. Further intervention, using the DTR, focused on the patient's cognitive distortions of minimization, disqualifying the positive, and all-or-nothing thinking.

A second problem identified was Mr. D.'s tendency to engage in verbalizations and thinking characterized by derogatory self-labeling. For example, he regularly had thoughts like "feeling depressed shows I have a weak character." He also flagellated himself for feeling anything less than happy around other family members. Once again, we decreased the severity of this problem using the DTR. With regular work, he saw that feeling depressed proved nothing about his character (magnification and labeling), but rather that he was human and depressed, and that there was no reason he should feel any particular emotions around his family. They accepted him regardless of how he felt. Although by objective standards the patient's mood was improved, the pain associated with the circulatory trouble in his lower extremities increased during the second half of treatment. In spite of active medical intervention, he became less mobile, necessitating a change to an every-other-week schedule after the 12th meeting. Several weeks had passed under this arrangement when the patient's son called to say Mr. D. had fallen and fractured his hip. More important, Mr. D. had been hiding a drinking problem from his therapist. Apparently, he had been drinking alone in the evenings, although he denied drinking at the time of his fall.

Therapy shifted to home visits while the patient convalesced. Initially, much work was directed at confronting Mr. D.'s denial of his drinking problem. This denial was fueled by Mr. D.'s belief that only "bad" or "weak" people abused alcohol and that he would be hated by his family if he admitted to such a problem. After doing numerous DTRs between sessions, he eventually accepted himself as a person with a drinking problem rather than a "bad" person, and saw that others accepted him as well. The issue also proved to be fruitful in terms of highlighting and addressing the approval needs that had prevented him from discussing his drinking problem with his therapist. Strategies for relapse prevention (Marlatt and Gordon 1985) were

15

discussed and included plans for continued treatment in a 12-step program (similar to Alcoholics Anonymous).

The relapse prevention strategy was timely because, during a medical follow-up appointment, Mr. D. was diagnosed with mild emphysema. Although he initially interpreted this as "the end," the patient was soon able to view his problem more reasonably. He immediately quit smoking and the relapse prevention strategies were applied to both his addictions. Meanwhile, his hip healed rapidly and, although his general physical condition led to a diminution in his level of functioning, Mr. D. was able to express appropriate feelings of loss combined with an attitude of adaptation. By the 20th session, he was able to drive himself to the center with little discomfort and felt quite proud about this. At termination (session 22) his depression had remitted, leaving only residual symptoms. At a 3-month follow-up, Mr. D. was very pleased to report no recurrence of his drinking or smoking problems or of his depression. He had become more active in several local senior organizations and felt that he could maintain himself "on an even keel" in the months ahead.

FOR WHOM DOES COGNITIVE-BEHAVIORAL THERAPY WORK BEST?

In our experience, the majority of older persons in affective distress can derive at least some benefit from a course of CB therapy, which normally consists of 15 to 20 sessions of about an hour's duration (Thompson et al. 1987). We have conducted several outcome studies over the past 10 years and have found that 75% of patients show either full remission or definite improvement by the end of their outpatient therapy. In our studies, improvement has been defined as a change in the clinically rated diagnosis to a less severe level and improved self-report of symptoms on a measure such as the Beck Depression Inventory (Beck et al. 1961).

Our research has also indicated several important findings that should be kept in mind when deciding whether or not to use this therapeutic modality with a given patient. First, the greatest success comes in treatment of reactive depressions for which a clear precipitant can be determined and much of the depression can be seen as a response to this specific event or situation. Our most recent study (Thompson et al. 1987) has shown that this factor is strongly linked to full remission of major depression. We have also noted that patients with chronic depression or with a depressive episode superimposed on a dysthymia of long duration can be treated effectively as long as the more modest goals are set and the general aim is for improved affective status rather than complete remission of the disorder. In other words, a chronically depressed older patient who complains of more or less lifetime dissatisfaction can be helped by selecting a specific problem or source of distress in the here and now that can be addressed in CB terms, such as relationship difficulties or a low level of engagement in pleasant activities. Second, in our current ongoing research, we are finding that extending therapy for 30 to 40 sessions can be helpful when treating the chronic patient. It seems to take them longer to "get going" in therapy and to make modifications that lead to discernible improvement in mood. This practice of extending the number of treatment sessions is consistent with recommendations by other CB therapists (e.g., Young 1990; A. Beck, March 1986, personal communication) who have extended this treatment modality to work with patients who are suffering from an Axis II personality disorder as well as depression or anxiety.

Regarding our experience with the use of CB in older patients with personality disorder, we have found that about half respond very well (often after a more protracted course of treatment) and about half do not seem to improve much (Thompson et al. 1988). It may be that even longer term CB therapy is needed to effect significant change in the latter 50%. The same general statistic applies to patients evidencing strong signs of endogenous depression: about half respond very well to CB therapy alone without added psychotropic medication and about half require either the addition of medication or other modalities, such as ECT, or require therapy of longer duration than would be typical in CB practice. However, with patience and persistence on the part of both client and therapist, improvement, at least to some degree, in symptomatic distress will generally occur.

There are few older patients for whom we would say that at least a trial of CB therapy is definitely contraindicated. We have used this method of therapy even with mildly demented patients (e.g., Alzheimer's victims or post-stroke patients not evidencing severe cognitive impairment) and have found it to be successful in improving mood and encouraging adaptive functioning (Teri and Gallagher-Thompson, in press; Thompson et al. 1989). Patients whom we have not generally treated with CB have been those in acute suicidal crisis or in very severe depression (e.g., requiring inpatient hospitalization or ECT), and those with severe cognitive impairment. In general, however, we have found that most other factors should be viewed as part and parcel of the presenting situation, but not necessarily as "red flags" (e.g., the presence of endogenous features or an Axis II diagnosis).

17

CONCLUSION

We hope that this chapter has provided sufficiently detailed information to encourage the reader to consider CB therapy with older adults who suffer from affective disorders. It is clear that many outpatients suffering from depression can benefit from this approach. Given that psychotropic medication is often contraindicated in older persons or is simply not tolerated, CB therapy can be a welcome addition to the clinician's armamentarium for the treatment of affective disorders in this population. Very little is known about the efficacy of this modality in dealing with elderly depressed inpatients. Based on a recent study of young and middleaged adults evaluating the effects of CB therapy as an adjunct to the "usual" inpatient treatment program, the argument could be made that CB therapy might conceivably decrease relapse in elderly inpatients following release from the hospital setting (Miller et al. 1989). Clinical experience also suggests that there may be instances when the combination of medication and CB therapy will accelerate the rate of short-term improvement in patients who show little change over a 3- or 4-month course of treatment. However, the use of CB therapy and psychotropic medication together is an area that is in need of much further study in both inpatient and outpatient samples. At present there are few research data to clarify when this combination would be preferable to either form of treatment alone.

REFERENCES

Beck AT, Rush AJ, Shaw BF, et al: Cognitive Therapy of Depression. New York, Guilford, 1979

Beck AT, Emery G, Greenberg RL: Anxiety Disorders and Phobias. New York, Basic Books, 1985

Burns DD: Feeling Good: The New Mood Therapy. New York, Signet, 1980

Burns DD: The Feeling Good Handbook: Using the New Mood Therapy in Everyday Life. New York, William Morrow, 1989

Butler RN, Gastel B: Hearing and age. Ann Otol Rhinol Laryngol 43:676–682, 1979

Emery G: Cognitive therapy with the elderly, in New Directions in Cognitive Therapy. Edited by Emery G, Hollon SD, Bedrosian RC, et al. New York, Guilford, 1981, pp 84–98

Gallagher D, Thompson LW: Depression in the Elderly: A Behavioral Treatment Manual. Los Angeles, University of Southern California Press, 1981

Gallagher D, Thompson LW: Cognitive therapy for depression in the elderly: a promising model for treatment and research, in Depression and Aging:

Causes, Care, and Consequences. Edited by Breslau LD, Haug MR. New York, Springer, 1983, pp 168–192

Goldfried MR, Davison GC: Clinical Behavior Therapy. New York, Holt Rinehart & Winston, 1976

Hussian RA, Davis RL: Responsive Care: Behavioral Interventions With Elderly Persons. Champaign, IL, Research Press, 1985

Kanfer FH, Grimm LG: Managing clinical change: a process model of therapy. Behav Modif 4:419–444, 1980

Lewinsohn PM, Munoz RF, Youngren MA, et al: Control Your Depression, Rev Edition. New York, Prentice-Hall, 1986

Marlatt A, Gordon J (eds): Relapse Prevention: Maintenance Strategies in Addictive Behavior Change. New York, Guilford, 1985

McMullin RE: Handbook of Cognitive Therapy Techniques. New York, Norton, 1986

Miller IW, Norman WH, Keitner GI: Cognitive-behavioral treatment of depressed inpatients: six- and twelve-month follow-up. J Am Psychiatry 146:1274–1279, 1989

Pankrantz L, Kofoed L: The assessment and treatment of geezers. JAMA 259:1228–1229, 1988

Stelnick G, Thompson JK: Eating disorders in the elderly. Behavior Therapist 12:7–9, 1989

Teri L, Gallagher-Thompson D: Cognitive behavioral interventions for treatment of depression in Alzheimer's patients. Gerontologist (in press)

Thompson LW, Davies R, Gallagher D, et al: Cognitive therapy with older adults. Clinical Gerontologist 5:245–279, 1986

Thompson LW, Gallagher D, Steinmetz-Breckenridge J: Comparative effectiveness of psychotherapies for depressed elders. J Consult Clin Psychol 55:385–390, 1987

Thompson LW, Gallagher D, Czirr R: Personality disorder and outcome in the treatment of late-life depression. J Geriatr Psychiatry 21:133–146, 1988

Thompson LW, Wagner B, Zeiss A, et al: Cognitive/Behavioral Therapy With Early Stage Alzheimer's Patients: An Exploratory View of the Utility of This Approach (DHHS Publ No ADM-89-1569). Washington, DC, U.S. Dept of Health and Human Services, 1989

Troll LE: Early and Middle Adulthood, 2nd Edition. Monterey, CA, Brooks/Cole, 1985

Willis SL: Toward an educational psychology of the older adult learner: intellectual and cognitive bases, in Handbook of Psychology and Aging. Edited by Birren J, Schaie KW. New York, Van Nostrand Reinhold, 1985, pp 818–847

Young J: Cognitive Therapy for Personality Disorders: A Schema-Focused Approach. Sarasota, FL: Professional Resources Exchange, 1990

Chapter Two

SEX THERAPY WITH OLDER PATIENTS

Helen Singer Kaplan, M.D., Ph.D.

Although it is widely believed that getting older entails the loss of sexuality, in actual fact sex is one of the last biological functions to fall prey to the aging process. There are countless older people who are retired, who are grandparents, or who are wearing hearing aids or reading glasses who still enjoy making love.

A number of surveys of sexual behavior in the aging population have been conducted in recent years (Brecher 1984; George and Weiler 1981; Palmore 1970, 1974; Starr and Weiner 1981; Todarello and Boscia 1985; Weizman and Hart 1987). These studies, which involved tens of thousands of men and women between the ages of 50 and 100, are unanimous in their findings that the majority of healthy older people remain sexually active on a regular basis into advanced old age. According to all studies conducted to date (Table 2-1), close to 70% of men and women in their seventies who are free of disease and are not taking medications with sexual side effects have sex about once a week.

The remainder, as well as a large additional group of older men and women who have minor medical problems, become totally dysfunctional because they cannot handle the biological slowdown in their sexual responses. These patients are frequently amenable to sex therapy, if that treatment is modified to accommodate the age-related changes in sexual response and the special vulnerabilities of the elderly.

AGE-RELATED CHANGES IN SEXUAL FUNCTIONING

To remain sexually functional, aging persons must adapt successfully to certain specific age-related changes in their sexual responses.

Table 2-1. Sex and the aging process: summary of recent studies

Study	Year	*n*	Age range (years)	Outcome
Kinsey et al. 1948 Kinsey et al. 1953	1948 1953	212 m 152 f	51–90 51–80	70% of couples are sexually active at age 70 on a regular basis. The average frequency over age 70 is 0.3 times a week.
Masters and Johnson 1966, 1970	1966, 1970	150 m 212 f	50–90	Found men and women in all age groups who remained sexually active on a regular basis.
Palmore 1970, 1974 (Duke University Longitudinal Study)	1953–1965 1968– present	250 m and f 502 m and f	60–90 45–69	70% of physically healthy couples have regular intercourse at age 68. In some cases, the frequency of sexual intercourse had increased.
Starr and Weiner 1981	1981	280 m 520 f	60–91	80% of total sample (m and f) are sexually active; 50% have sex on a regular basis, and, of these, 50% have intercourse at least once a week.
Brecher et al. 1984	1984	4,200 m and f	50–93	79% of men and 65% of women aged 70–91 are sexually active on a regular basis; 58% of men and 50% of women have sex every week.
All studies combined	1948–present	6,478 m and f	50–93	The majority of physically healthy men and women remain sexually active on a regular basis into their 9th decade.

Note. m = males. f = females.

It is important for the clinician who works with older patients to be knowledgeable about these and to understand their role in the pathogenesis of sexual disorders of the elderly.

The aging process affects men and women differently and differs in its impact on the three phases of the sexual response cycle: desire, excitement, and orgasm. In males, sexual desire peaks at age 17, then gradually declines; the female sex drive peaks at age 40, then begins to decline. In males and females the effects of age on sexual desire are variable after age 50: some men and women maintain a high level of sexual desire until their 80s and 90s; the sex drive of others declines significantly after the menopausal years. Testosterone is a factor influencing the level of sexual desire in both genders.

In the excitement phase, older men require increased and concomitant physical (genital) and psychic (erotic) stimulation in order to attain and maintain erections because the ability to have spontaneous erections declines and penile sensitivity decreases. Erections become less firm (Wagner and Green 1981), but remain rigid enough for penetration throughout old age. The length of time an erection can be maintained decreases with age and erections become progressively more vulnerable to the physiologic concomitants of emotional stress and anxiety (Kaplan 1989). Some men, as they age, experience a progressively longer delay in their ability to regain a lost erection even when they do not ejaculate (the paradoxical refractory period) (Masters and Johnson 1970). In older women the vagina tends to become dry and atrophic after menopause because of estrogen deficiency. Also, the vaginas of parous women can become stretched and lax due to rectocoele and cystocoele.

In the orgasm phase the refractory period for men lengthens significantly with age, from a few minutes at age 17 to a few days at 70. In females orgasm is not appreciably affected by age, so that women remain potentially multi-orgastic throughout life.

In sum, human sexual response does not disappear with age, though it does change in significant ways. These changes make men more dependent on women, physically and emotionally. More specifically, as the aging male loses his ability to have spontaneous erections and as his penile responsiveness declines, he needs his partners to supply him with the additional physical stimulation of his genitalia, which he now requires to attain and maintain his erection. Furthermore, since his ability to function becomes increasingly vulnerable to the effects of anxiety, with its concomitant adrenergic surge, the older man also becomes more dependent on his partner's unqualified emotional support and acceptance of his current level of functioning.

The aging woman faces different changes. In contrast to the male, her sex drive may remain high, and her ability to have orgasms endures, but she loses the bloom of her youthful physical attractiveness and must compensate for this with attractive personal qualities. Also, like the penis, the vaginal physiology undergoes senile changes as women age, and the vagina consequently becomes a less effective sexual organ. Women who have borne children may suffer from loss of vaginal muscle tone and stretching of the introitus, with the result that their partners feel less penile stimulation on coital thrusting. Post-menopausal women who do not receive estrogen replacement experience another problem. Their vaginas tend to become dry and tight and lose a certain erotic aroma, which makes lovemaking less exciting and intromission more difficult for their partners.

ADAPTATION VERSUS DYSFUNCTION

Since 1970, we have conducted highly detailed evaluations of the sexual functioning and behaviors of almost 500 patients with sexual complaints who were 50 years or older or whose partners were in that age group. Our population included couples who became totally dysfunctional, although they had only minor age-related changes in their physical capacity, and some who remained active in the face of considerable organic deficit. The patients described herein were seen by the author and her associates at the Human Sexuality Program of the Payne-Whitney Clinic of the New York Hospital–Cornell Medical Center and at their private practice group in Manhattan.

These extensive, in-depth clinical observations have made it clear that couples who are able to maintain their sexual functioning, despite significant age-related physical impairments, share a number of characteristics. First, they enjoy harmonious, intimate, communicative relationships which include a commitment to each other's well-being and sexual pleasure; second, the partners are free enough of serious sexual and neurotic conflicts and have enough self-esteem to feel entitled to good sex; third, they are open and nonjudgmental in their sexual attitudes.

Loving older couples who are conflict-free about sexual pleasure and highly committed and creative in their efforts to remain sexually active successfully adapt to age-related changes intuitively and imperceptibly. They accept the slowdown of their sexual responses in the same way as they do their presbyopia or their presbycussis—as a natural part of getting older and without overreacting or blaming their partners. Although his erections are a little softer and her vagina is a little dryer, these intimate couples do not avoid sex, because they are secure enough sexually and trust each other sufficiently to risk an occasional "failure."

Although it may not be her preference, the wife agrees, without making a power struggle out of it, to have sex in the morning when her elderly husband's erectile capacity is at its peak. She does not take the absence of his spontaneous erections during foreplay as a personal rejection, but lovingly supplies him, without being asked, with more intense penile stimulation. She may try oral or manual techniques to help his erections. Rather than objecting, she encourages the use of erotica (if this is compatible with the couple's value system) and she uses lubricants prior to getting into bed with him (so as not to create a stressful interruption) to protect her more fragile genitalia and to make penetration easier for him.

If the woman's vagina is lax, the couple uses concomitant manual stimulation or coital positions with the woman's legs closed to provide more penile friction. The man accepts these changes and accommodates to them without negative comment, while she, also silently, accepts her aging partner's diminishing "staying power." He, again without being asked, takes more time with foreplay and concentrates on giving his partner pleasure with manual or oral stimulation of her genitalia to compensate for the briefer periods of vaginal penetration. He is extra attentive to his post-menopausal wife, and makes certain that she feels that she is still attractive to him. Above all, neither ever threatens the other with inappropriate performance demands nor with criticisms or put-downs of the other's desirability or sexuality.

These flexible, conflict-free couples remain sexually active in the face of a considerable biological slowdown. This level of sexual activity does not occur, however, if the partners are ambivalent about remaining sexual or about each other. If the sexual slowdown occurs in a setting of latent marital hostility or if it taps into pre-existing sexual conflicts or if the couple is inflexible in their sexual behavior because of culturally programmed sexual guilts and inhibitions, serious sexual problems can develop. Such problems usually take the form of impotence, loss of sexual desire, and sexual avoidance.

The following case vignette illustrates some common issues in the pathogenesis and the treatment of sexual dysfunction in the elderly.

Mr. S., a 68-year-old highly successful corporate attorney, and his wife, an attractive, stylishly dressed 62-year-old woman, presented with a complaint of impotence and low sexual frequency. The couple had not made love in 4 months. Both were extremely distressed about their sexual difficulty and were pessimistic, because of the husband's age, about the possibility of improvement.

The couple had been married for 3 years. Mrs. S. had been divorced and had three grown children from a previous marriage. Mr. S. was a widower. He had been married to his first wife for 40 years and the couple had raised two children. The first Mrs. S. had died 5 years earlier, after a painful 3-year struggle with cancer. The marriage had been a harmonious and traditional one. The previous Mrs. S. had been her husband's first and only sexual partner and they had functioned well until she became ill. After that, the couple stopped having sex. Mr. S. had not had sexual relations with a partner nor had he masturbated during the 3 years of his wife's terminal illness and for the year after her death, until he met his present wife.

When the couple first became lovers, they had a few sexual encounters during which he had been able to penetrate, although he had ejaculated almost instantly. However, they both found the other very attractive and believed that their sexual relationship would improve after their marriage. Instead, it got worse.

Mr. S. desired his wife but he was somewhat intimidated by her and felt absolutely paralyzed by his performance anxiety. Mrs. S. was a demanding partner. In addition to complaining that her husband did not achieve a spontaneous erection when they got into bed together, she also refused to let him stimulate her manually, only wanting the "real thing." She was most unenthusiastic about "helping him out" with penile stimulation and she denied his request for morning sex. He tried his best to accede to her wishes, but on the one occasion when he had managed to arouse himself by rubbing his genitalia against her body, he had ejaculated rapidly with a flaccid penis before entering her vagina and she had shouted out "Oh no!" Since that time, 4 months ago, he had been avoiding sex.

He admitted that on those few occasions early in their relationship when he did achieve penetration, he had felt very little sensation and had ejaculated rapidly because of his fear of losing his erection. After these experiences he felt a growing apprehension about his ability to function sexually and about his capacity to satisfy his wife, which, of course, ensured that he would fail.

ASSESSING PHYSICAL LIMITATIONS AND RESERVES

The initial step in evaluating a couple such as Mr. and Mrs. S. involves the assessment of their physical limitations and reserves. "Silent" disease states that affect sexual functioning, such as diabetes and prolactin-secreting adenomas, and conditions requiring medications that affect sexual functioning, such as hypertension, become more prevalent as people age. For this reason, the physical aspects of the evaluation are especially important with older patients. If the clinical picture raises any question of organicity, it is our practice carefully to screen older patients with sexual complaints for possible organic problems. We routinely conduct a physical examination of the genitalia for patients complaining of dyspareunia and a comprehensive hormone screening for those with low sexual desire and delayed orgasms. Our screening test includes balancing levels of serum testosterone, estradiol, progesterone, prolactin, leutinizing hormone, follicle-stimulating hormone, and, for men only, acid phosphatase. Lipid and thyroid profiles may be added as indicated.

Our pre-sex therapy workup of men with erectile complaints often includes additional studies such as nocturnal penile tumescence (NPT) monitoring. When indicated, we also arrange for papaverine and duplex studies of the penile circulation, penile neurophysiological studies, and cavernosography. If any abnormality is detected, the patient is referred to the appropriate specialist for further evaluation and treatment.

Using this diagnostic format, we have detected organic problems in approximately 50% of our patients over the age of 50, although the impairments were severe enough to preclude sexual functioning in only 10% of our patient population.

In our assessment of Mr. and Mrs. S., it turned out that both husband and wife had minor physical problems with which they could not cope. Mr. S. was found to have a minor impairment of his penile circulation on the papaverine and duplex studies. However, his NPT results indicated that he was still capable of achieving fairly good erections during the early morning hours. Mrs. S.'s vaginal examination revealed a moderate degree of cystocoele and rectocoele.

PATHOGENESIS

A detailed exploration of this couple's current sexual experience revealed that the immediate cause of their failure to adapt to their minor age-related physical deficits was their disastrous sexual interaction (Kaplan 1979). This created insurmountable performance pressure for the husband and little if any erotic gratification for the wife. On a deeper psychological level, to Mr. S., who had been reared in a devout Catholic home, sex was still somehow "dirty," while on her part, Mrs. S. had never overcome her neurotic conflicts about romantic success. In addition, both were extremely sensitive to rejection, and their sensitivities were not only a gratifying point of contact between them and also a source of difficulty. These issues were not of a magnitude to have impaired their sexual functioning when they were younger, but were now interfering with their ability to adapt to the age-related changes in their sexual capacities. Mr. S. felt like a failure because he expected himself to perform as he had in his younger years, with spontaneous erections and the ability to continue thrusting until his partner had climaxed. Since he himself did not accept the limitations imposed by age, it did not occur to him to expect his partner to do so.

This patient was unable to make himself comfortable with his new wife in their sexual encounters for several reasons. He was neither secure enough in his masculinity, nor sufficiently trusting with his wife to overcome his performance fears. These fears had their origins in the long years of abstinence during his first wife's illness. His insecurity was amplified by his sensing the slight decline in erectile capacity that had occurred during this time. In addition, the guilt about erotic pleasure that was a legacy of his early puritanical upbringing blocked him from communicating effectively with his wife. Thus, he was far too guilt-stricken and uncomfortable to be able to ask her for the genital stimulation which he physically needed and for the oral sex which he secretly craved.

Mrs. S. was unable to enjoy sex with her husband. Her sexual preference had always been to be the recipient of ardent lovemaking by a highly aroused, passionate man. Her new husband's sexual difficulties and his performance anxieties simply "turned her off." She had no patience for stimulating him and she was too emotionally vulnerable herself to be the active, supportive, encouraging partner he needed. She had always been a rejection-sensitive woman, and her anxieties had been heightened by her post-menopausal status. She personalized her husband's potency problem and felt threatened by it. She took his difficulty as a sign that age had robbed her of her power to attract men. In her attempts to reassure herself, she became even more sexually demanding of him.

She was also angry at her husband for having pressured her into signing a prenuptial agreement that she regarded as extremely unfair and unfavorable. And on a deeper level, of which she was only dimly aware, there was also a passive-aggressive element in her inflexibility in the bedroom.

SEX THERAPY WITH OLDER PATIENTS

Sex therapy employs an integrated amalgam of behavioral interventions to modify the immediate, currently operating causes of sexual disorders and active, psychodynamically oriented psychotherapeutic methods to deal with the couple's deeper emotional and marital problems (Kaplan 1974, 1979, 1987). With some modifications, we have found this method ideally suited to treatment of the sexual problems in older men and women.

The first step in sex therapy with older patients and couples consists of reconceptualizing their problems realistically and helping them to accept their limitations, while maintaining a positive, optimistic attitude about their remaining capacities. We attempt to promote the feeling that "while much was taken, much endures."

After the couple has come to terms with these realities, sexual techniques designed to reduce the anxieties impairing their sexual reflexes and others that compensate for each partner's particular organic deficits are prescribed for the couple to conduct in the privacy of their home. At the same time, the fears and resistances that are often mobilized by these new, sometimes previously avoided and often threatening erotic and intimate experiences are dealt with in the office sessions with the therapist in an active, psychodynamically oriented manner.

For example, Mr. and Mrs. S. were informed that each had an actual, rather common physical problem. In both cases the problem was minor but had escalated into a serious sexual dysfunction because of their emotional reactions. The couple was reassured that these physical problems would not prevent them from having a good sex life together, providing they were committed to accomplishing this and were willing to change their sexual techniques.

Mr. S.'s NPT record was reviewed with the couple to demonstrate objectively to both spouses that he retained sufficient erectile capacity to function under the proper conditions. The laboratory evidence that his physical capability to have erections was significantly better in the mornings helped to defuse the couple's struggle about morning sex. The concomitant finding that Mrs. S. had some vaginal stretching and laxness gave credence to Mr. S.'s complaints of diminished sensation on penetration. The couple was advised that this difficulty was slight and that Mr. S. was overreacting to it. At the same time, they were assured that if sexual therapy did not help with this issue, a minor surgical procedure could correct the problem.

Behavioral Aspects of Treatment

We have developed different and specific behavioral protocols to treat each of the eight sexual dysfunctions listed in DSM-III (American Psychiatric Association 1980). These protocols consist of therapeutically structured sexual interactions which have been described in detail elsewhere (Kaplan 1974, 1979, 1987; Masters and Johnson

1970). These "homework assignments" are modified and individualized to compensate for older patients' emotional and physical limitations and to maximize their remaining capacities. The following are some examples of behavioral assignments that we have found useful with patients over 50.

The sensate focus (SF) exercises (Masters and Johnson 1970), which are excellent for diminishing the performance anxiety to which the older male is now more vulnerable, are often indicated, with some modifications, for older couples. Assignments that expose the elderly person to new levels of physical and emotional intimacy are frequently used to modify the old routines that no longer work and to introduce the greater degree of sexual flexibility that is now needed to overcome the physical limitations imposed by age. Tasks geared toward the freeing up of sexual fantasy and the encouragement of sharing erotica can often help to supply both the extra sensual stimulation and the necessary distraction from performance anxiety that may help an older couple to remain functional. Sexual techniques that entail more tender and gentle lovemaking and the use of lubricants are frequently prescribed to protect the post-menopausal woman's more fragile genitalia.

Physical stimulation of the genitalia is emphasized for both partners. We often help women to overcome their resistance to providing their partners with more penile stimulation with oral and manual techniques. This is helpful to make up for the loss of sensation which occurs because of the relaxation of the aging woman's vaginal muscles combined with the aging man's decreasing penile sensitivity. Just as frequently, we devise assignments that are designed to improve the husband's lovemaking skill. We work on this technique of stimulating his wife's genitalia, especially her clitoris, orally and manually, to make up for his softer erections, his longer refractory period, and the shorter period of penile thrusting that he is now able to provide for her. As a general rule, we attempt to shift the couple's objective in lovemaking away from lengthy penetration and toward the exchange of sensuous pleasure in other ways. This deemphasis on coitus and the encouragement of experimenting with alternative forms of gratification can provide more pleasure for the aging woman and reduce the performance pressure for the aging man.

Often, the initial behavioral assignment for impotent patients is the SF-I exercise, in which intercourse is proscribed and the couple take turns caressing each other's bodies (Masters and Johnson 1970). This is an excellent tactic for reducing performance anxiety and often produces erections in younger men. Since this would not be the expected result in a man of Mr. S.'s age, my first assignment for this couple was SF-II (Kaplan 1979, 1987).

During this exercise the partners also caress each other's bodies sensuously. In addition, they take turns stimulating each other's genitals. This is done only in a teasing way, which allows the exchange of pleasurable sensations between the partners without the imposition of any performance requirements. Utilizing this technique, Mr. S. achieved an erection that would have been sufficient for penetration. He and I were both pleased, but Mrs. S. "did not like" the assignment.

The next behavioral step was to repeat the SF-II procedure to orgasm. The couple was asked to use lubricants and to take turns stimulating each other's genitalia. Mr. S. was asked to close his eyes and focus on his favorite erotic fantasy while his wife was stimulating him in order to teach him to "tune out" his performance anxiety. She was advised to focus on the pleasurable erotic clitoral sensations when it was her turn to "receive." This worked very well for him, but not for her. He achieved an erection and had an enjoyable orgasm. Instead of feeling encouraged by this visible evidence of her husband's sexual capacity, Mrs. S. was upset. She was unable to feel any pleasure in response to his caresses and she objected to his "messy" semen.

The next assignment entailed the couple's experimenting with oral sex. While she complied with the assignment, Mrs. S. only went through the motions and managed to sabotage the treatment process by grimacing with disgust and making a big show of taking a pubic hair out of her mouth. Mrs. S. was obviously resisting therapy.

Psychodynamic Aspects of Treatment

When they are young and sexually vigorous, men and women can often function despite the remnants of the antisexual conditioning of their childhood, despite some degree of sexual insecurity, despite the existence of some unresolved intrapsychic conflict, and despite the presence of a certain level of latent marital hostility. However, as people age and as their sexuality becomes more fragile, all of their old problems tend to resurface and to create sexual difficulties as well as resistances to treatment. The following are some of the deeper issues that commonly mobilize resistances in elderly patients undergoing sexual therapy.

Men's increasing sexual dependence on women. The assignments which are prescribed for older couples often entail the wife's taking a more active role in lovemaking, while the husband learns to accept a more passive or more "receiving" position. Not surprisingly, such unfamiliar or previously avoided experiences and role shifts can evoke intense anxiety in either or both partners.

The older man's greater dependence on his partner can rekindle old, buried feelings of ambivalence toward women in men who have never completely gotten over their problems with their mothers. Sometimes when such men find themselves once again in a dependent position, they displace the rage that they once felt toward their mothers onto their current partners. This is especially likely to occur in men who saw their mothers as rejecting or controlling or overprotective. Not surprisingly, the husband's unwarranted hostility does not inspire his wife's enthusiastic cooperation in bed. According to a psychodynamic formulation, such "parental" transferences are indicative of unresolved oedipal and preoedipal issues, which are common "deeper" etiologic factors in the sexual problems of the elderly and are sources of resistance to the process of treatment.

Erotica and fantasy. The introduction of erotica and sexual fantasies is another common source of resistance to treatment. Rejection-sensitive wives are often threatened by the therapist's suggestion that their husbands attempt to "tune out" their performance anxieties and obsessions by focusing on a sexual fantasy. If the woman is emotionally fragile, she may misinterpret the fact that her partner can be aroused by the image of somebody else as a painful, personal rejection. There are several cases in our files in which a poor therapeutic outcome could be directly attributed to our inability to resolve the wife's resistance to erotica and our failure to get her to see that her aging husband's desire for fantasy was not a personal insult to her, but rather his attempt to avoid disappointing her by losing his erection.

The therapist's suggestion that a couple try erotic videotapes or books and encouragement of fantasy can also mobilize resistances in conventional individuals whose religious or traditional backgrounds have conditioned them to feel guilty and ashamed about their sexual feelings and fantasies, especially if these vary from the norm.

These inhibitions must be worked through before a person can embrace the therapist's "permission" to enjoy their sexuality and to engage in previously taboo sexual behaviors, such as oral sex or the adjunctive use of fantasy. A strong, positive transference with the therapist and an identification with his or her more liberal sexual values is the key to the resolution of such "cultural" resistances.

32

Marital hostilities. Not infrequently, age-related sexual changes evoke latent marital hostilities and resistance to treatment. The therapist's inability to resolve these is the greatest single cause of treatment failure in the sex therapy of older couples.

In one common scenario, the aging man's growing sexual dependency gives his wife, who may have felt helpless, angry, and at the mercy of her controlling, aggressive, difficult husband throughout the early years of their marriage, the perfect opportunity to get even. Such passive-aggressive wives usually do not directly refuse the sexual requests of their husbands. Instead, they act out their anger in various and subtle ways. Some succeed in "castrating" their husbands simply by withholding their acceptance and support. Others express their anger by their passivity and unresponsiveness in bed, which can be devastating for a man who is proud of his lovemaking powers. Still others manage to undermine their partner's sexual confidence with criticisms of his sexual functioning or by making inappropriate performance demands.

It is equally common for an angry husband to punish his wife for his own sexual decline by neglecting or rejecting her. We often see men who have been in long-standing power struggles with their difficult, controlling wives withdraw from them emotionally and avoid sex when their own sexuality becomes more fragile. These passive-aggressive men do not openly communicate their sexual needs and concerns to their wives. Rather, they create the impression that the sexual problem is her fault. Such a cruel pattern of detachment can last for years, leaving the vulnerable, post-menopausal wife feeling rejected and devastated.

Many older couples who seek help to restore their sexual functioning have been too angry at each other for too long to be able to commit themselves to or benefit from a treatment that aims to increase their pleasure together. Such adversarial couples require prior conjoint counseling in order to resolve their marital conflicts before it makes sense to deal with their sexual symptoms.

Overcoming resistance. There are two keys to the successful restoration of sexual functioning in older patients. One is the introduction of appropriate compensatory and therapeutic sexual technique and realistic and constructive attitudes. These are in many respects similar to the adaptive behaviors that are spontaneously arrived at by those fortunate older individuals described earlier, those who remain sexually functional into advanced old age. But behavioral and cognitive interventions, no matter how astute they may be, are usually not sufficient by themselves to cure these patients. The real art of psychosexual therapy with this population involves the therapist's sensitive and totally unambivalent support of the older couple's sexuality and his or her ability to diffuse the resistances that are typically mobilized by the treatment process.

Our active, psychodynamically oriented method of resolving or "bypassing" resistances in brief sexual therapy has been described in other publications (Kaplan 1974, 1979, 1986). In essence, it entails the confrontation and exploration, on progressively "deeper" levels of consciousness, of the underlying unconscious intrapsychic conflicts and the hidden marital struggles that militate against successful sexual functioning and also mobilize obstacles to treatment. The energetic therapeutic interventions that characterize this method typically disrupt the resisting partner's psychological defenses and expose his or her vulnerability. For this reason, the active confrontations must always be balanced by the equally active emotional support of both partners and of the positive elements of the couple's relationship.

The relentless confrontations and resistances create crises that offer both hazards and opportunities (Kaplan 1979). The danger, of course, is that the therapist will be unable to resolve or "detour around" the patient's resistances and so the couple will fail to improve.

But these therapeutic crises can also open up the opportunity to extend the benefits of treatment beyond the target goal of simply restoring sexual functioning. This is because the resistances have their origins in the couple's pre-existing, latent intrapsychic conflicts and in the buried difficulties in their relationship. In many cases, these problems have troubled these individuals or impaired their functioning in areas apart from the sexual sphere. These issues are lured to the surface in the form of resistances during the process of psychosexual therapy, and this material then becomes available for therapeutic exploration.

Although many people whose sexual symptoms improve in response to sex therapy show no evidence of functioning better in other areas, it is also not unusual for a patient to gain insight into and to resolve, at least in part, long-standing success and commitment conflicts. Also, at the termination of sex therapy, there is often a visible improvement of a couple's sense of intimacy and a lessening of their hostilities. Such therapeutic bonuses are most often seen in the more complex cases, which require a good deal of psychodynamic exploration of resistance.

For example Mrs. S. was confronted by the therapist with her conflicts about improving her sexual relationship with her husband: "It seems part of you really wants to make this marriage work and to resolve your sexual problem. But another part of you seems ambivalent about this and appears to be sabotaging treatment."

The week following this interpretation, she brought in an anxiety-laden dream. The patient dreamed that she was still unmarried. She was frantically looking for a husband but could not find anyone. She felt despair that she would always be alone, while everyone else was coupled, and awoke in panic. She was greatly relieved to find her husband in bed beside her.

The dream was interpreted as a "reassurance dream" (Freud 1900) and as an "early warning" of impending psychic danger. I told Mrs. S. that her relief when she woke up and found her husband beside her probably meant that she did not really want to lose him. I further noted that her "unconscious" was warning her to stop being destructive to her marriage.

This interpretation proved to be ego-syntonic. The patient was eager for me to support the relationship and was not resistant to exploring her long-standing pattern of self-destructive behavior in romantic relationships. She began to recognize that throughout her life she had sabotaged herself either by picking men who had exploited her or by driving away those who would have been good partners. Signing a prenuptial agreement, which she now felt she could not live with, without having made the slightest attempt to negotiate was simply the latest example of how she had set things up to defeat herself.

We spent a brief time exploring the childhood roots of her compelling urge to "snatch defeat out of the jaws of victory." These discussions centered around her ambivalent relationship with her competitive, narcissistic, and alcoholic mother, whom she had futilely attempted to appease throughout her childhood. In her therapy sessions, she became aware that, by not having allowed herself to have a successful relationship with a desirable man, she had still been unconsciously complying with her mother's destructive wishes.

For his part, Mr. S. needed to overcome the long-standing sense of sexual guilt and inadequacy that had made him an anxious and unattractive partner. With the therapist's support he soon came to see himself in a more realistic light, as the desirable man he actually was.

We also worked to resolve the couple's struggle about money and control. Mr. S. had used his wealth in an attempt to protect himself from rejection and abandonment, which he greatly feared. On an unconscious level, he felt that no beautiful woman could love him solely "for himself." Only by the use of economic leverage could he ensure that his lovely wife would stay with him, despite what he saw as his sexual inadequacy. He came to realize how counterproductive his attempts to control her by means of money were, inasmuch as this merely infuriated and alienated her further. With these insights, the couple began to resolve their power struggle.

As their trust in each other and in their relationship grew, their commitment to each other deepened. He became less withholding with money and she became less withholding with sex. At the end of treatment the couple were having sex on a regular basis. Mrs. S. learned to overcome her avoidance of oral and manual stimulation of her husband's genitalia. She also came to accept his current level of sexual functioning, including his need for morning sex and his more rapid ejaculations.

Mrs. S. chose not to have a vaginoplasty at this time. Instead, the couple began to utilize sexual techniques that provided more stimulation for Mr. S. during coitus. On his part, Mr. S. learned to be a more confident, sensitive lover, which led to greater gratification for his wife.

PROGNOSIS

Too many clinicians, unaware that the loss of sexuality is not an inevitable aspect of aging, approach the sexual complaints of their older patients in a defeatist manner. When this attitude is found in conjunction with the countertransferentially determined tendency, common especially in younger therapists, to avoid acknowledging their parents' and grandparents' sexuality, it reduces the chances of a positive treatment outcome. Specifically, such negative attitudes militate against both the meticulous search for potentially treatable medical conditions and the vigorous disruption of the older patient's defenses and resistances, two of the most important ingredients in the successful outcome of sexual therapy.

Clinicians should be aware that, as a result of our increased understanding of the pathogenesis of sexual dysfunction in the elderly and the recent advances in sexual medicine that allow us to diagnose and treat an increasingly greater number of physical problems, sexual functioning can be restored or materially improved in a high proportion of elderly patients. The prognosis is especially good in those couples who had enjoyed a good sexual relationship prior to the onset of age-related changes in their sexual functioning.

The treatment of elderly patients with sexual problems can be extremely gratifying for the therapist because the restoration of sexual activity is often a tremendous gift to the older patient. Though it is widely believed that sex no longer matters as an individual gets older, the opposite is often true. Sex may become more important in a person's life with the passage of time because sexuality is among the last of the pleasure-giving biological processes to deteriorate. It is a potentially enduring source of emotional well-being at a time when more and more losses must be accepted and fewer and fewer gratifications remain available.

REFERENCES

American Psychiatric Association: Diagnostic and Statistical Manual of Mental Disorders, 3rd Edition. Washington, DC, American Psychiatric Association, 1980

Brecher EM, editors of Consumer Reports Books: Love, Sex and Aging. Boston, Little, Brown, 1984

Freud S: The interpretation of dreams (1900), in The Standard Edition of the Complete Psychological Works of Sigmund Freud, Vol IV, V. Translated and edited by Strachey J. London, Hogarth Press, 1962, pp 273–276

George LK, Weiler SJ: Sexuality in middle and late life. Arch Gen Psychiatry 38:919–923, 1981

Kaplan HS: The New Sex Therapy. New York, Brunner/Mazel, 1974

Kaplan HS: Disorders of Sexual Desire. New York, Brunner/Mazel, 1979

Kaplan HS: Sexual Aversion, Sexual Phobias, and Panic Disorder. New York, Brunner/Mazel, 1987

Kaplan HS: The concept of presbyrectia. International Journal of Impotence Research 1:16–21, 1989

Kinsey AC, Pomeroy WB, Martin CG: Sexual Behavior in the Human Male. Philadelphia, PA, Saunders, 1948

Kinsey AC, Pomeroy WB, Martin CG: Sexual Behavior in the Human Female. Philadelphia, PA, Saunders, 1953

Masters WB, Johnson VE: The Human Sexual Response. Boston, Little, Brown, 1966

Masters WB, Johnson VE: Human Sexual Inadequacy. Boston, Little, Brown, 1970

Palmore E (ed): Normal Aging. Durham, NC, Duke University Press, 1970

Palmore E (ed): Normal Aging, Vol II. Durham, NC, Duke University Press, 1974

Starr BD, Weiner MB: The Starr-Weiner Report on Sex and Sexuality in the Mature Years. New York, McGraw-Hill, 1981

Todarello O, Boscia FM: Sexuality in aging: a study of a group of 300 elderly men and women. J Endocrinol Invest 8 (suppl 2):123–129, 1985

Wagner G, Green R: Impotence. New York, Plenum, 1981

Weizman R, Hart J: Sexual behavior in healthy married elderly men. Arch Sex Behav 16:39–44, 1987

Chapter Three

CAREGIVERS OF PERSONS WITH CHRONIC ILLNESSES OR IMPAIRMENTS: STRATEGIES AND INTERVENTIONS

Kenneth Hepburn, Ph.D., Wayne Caron, M.A., and John R. Mach, Jr., M.D.

This chapter focuses on the important role that family members play in the care of chronically impaired older people and on how physicians and clinical teams can orient themselves to the caregiver to provide better patient care and to maintain the well-being of the family caregiver using a variety of therapeutic strategies. The chapter reflects the clinical experience of the Geriatric Research, Education, and Clinical Center (GRECC) at the Minneapolis Veterans Administration Medical Center, a multidisciplinary team with special interest in the evaluation and extended care of chronically ill and demented patients. The concerns and strategies of this team are appropriate for all chronic illnesses.

BACKGROUND

As we move toward the 21st century, economics and demography will influence clinical practice even more significantly than they have in the last decade. By the year 2000, national health care expenditures (public and private) will reach $1.5 trillion, with a tripling in annual per capita expenditures to $5,550. Nursing home costs are expected to parallel this threefold growth to $129 billion (HCFA 1987).

The Elderly as Heavy Users of Care Services

The elderly—those over 65 years of age, but particularly those over 85 years—will necessarily be targeted for efforts to contain national health care expenditures. In 1985, 6.2–6.5 million elderly persons were determined to be functionally impaired, i.e., to have some need for chronic assistance with Activities of Daily Living (ADL) or Instrumental Activities of Daily Living (IADL); 1.3–1.6 million needed help with almost all ADLs. About four-fifths of all functionally impaired persons live in the community; only one-fifth are institutionalized. The functionally impaired segment of the population is expected to increase as the number of elderly persons in the population increases. It is projected that in 2020 14.3 million elderly persons will have at least one ADL/IADL need; of these, about 4.2 million will need nursing home care (Comptroller General 1988), necessitating an expensive buildup of nursing home beds from the current supply of 1.6 million.

Older persons are more likely to experience chronic need. While about one-quarter of all persons 65 years of age and older report one or more ADL/IADL deficit, more than half of those 85 years and older report such deficits (USDHHS 1988). A significant portion of the chronically impaired elderly will be afflicted with dementing conditions, which also are more prevalent among those 85 years and older. Researchers' estimates of the number of moderately to severely demented persons range from 3.8 million by 2030 (Mortimer et al. 1985) to 7.3 million by 2040 (Cross and Gurland 1986).

The chronically impaired, including the demented, elderly are major users of health care and a major source of expenditures. Approximately 10% of the elderly incur 73% of the health care charges of this age group; 15% incur 81% of the charges (Garfinkel et al. 1988). The most important characteristic associated with high and frequent use of health care services is the presence of chronic conditions, including self-perception of poor health and restricted activity days (Garfinkel et al. 1988; Holloway et al. 1988).

Family Caregivers: Who Are They?

Family caregivers are the backbone of the chronic care system. The profiles of use and expense by the chronically ill and impaired would be virtually out of control were it not for the care provided by families and other unpaid caregivers. Despite changes in American social structure, the family remains a faithful provider of care to the chronically impaired. Research has consistently demonstrated that 80% of the in-home care needs of the chronically impaired elderly are met by families (Comptroller General 1977) and that for every person in a nursing home there are two just like him or her living in the community and being cared for by a family member (Brody et al. 1978; Shanas 1979). The most significant predictor of institutionalization is not the level of functioning of the impaired older person, but the presence or absence of a caregiving family member or friend (Brody et al. 1978; Johnson 1983). Family caregivers' effect on utilization extends beyond nursing home use: Coe and colleagues (1985) report a 7 to 30 times more frequent use of emergency room services by elderly persons without family than those with family in the area. The importance of family caregiving to the maintenance of elderly persons in the community and the containment of health care costs has led some to suggest that this form of care has become an implicit (but consciously unreimbursed) and major part of national health care policy (Brody et al. 1984).

Research provides a profile of family caregivers for the chronically impaired elderly. A national survey (Stone et al. 1987) found most caregivers are women (72%), typically older spouses not working outside the home, but one-third are daughters or daughters-in-law. Half of the male caregivers are spouses. These data also indicate that 80% of the caregivers provide care daily; caregivers provide an average of more than 4 hours of care per day; only 10% of the caregivers receive additional paid or unpaid help; and, while the majority of caregivers have provided help for 1–4 years, about 20% have done so for more than 5 years. Nor does caregiving occur in isolation from other demands: 21% of caregivers also have child care responsibilities, 20% report work-related conflicts, and another 9% have left their jobs. Caregiving responsibility tends to fall primarily on only one member of the family with others serving satellite functions (Horowitz 1985); sequential replacement by other family members occurs when the primary caregiver can no longer provide care (Johnson 1983). Caregivers expend their own resources to help provide care— in one recent study, $144 per month (Keenan et al. 1989).

The Impact of Caregiving on the Caregiver

The impact of caregiving on the caregivers is well documented. In particular, elderly spouse caregivers are understood to be at risk for mental and physical health problems themselves. Caregiving has a negative impact on self-reported health status, morale, mental health status, and perceived psychological distress and stress levels; it also produces higher than normal levels of psychotropic drug use (Eagles et al. 1987; George and Gwyther 1986; Pruchno and Potashnik 1989). Those who have provided care for a longer time report higher levels of morale and mental health than those who have been caregivers for a short time (Gilhooly 1984; Motenko 1989). Caregivers report lower overall life satisfaction and social participation (Haley et al. 1987a) and experience chronic fatigue, anger, depression, and family conflict (Rabins et al. 1982). Caregivers also report less use of health care services than the general population (Pruchno and Potashnik 1989).

Depression is a major problem for caregivers. Current estimates using DSM-III-R (American Psychiatric Association 1987) criteria put the prevalence of depression in the elderly at 1% for major depression, 2% for chronic depression, and another 4% for subclinical depression (Blazer et al. 1987). In contrast, a recent study of family caregivers of both demented and nondemented adults found that, according to Research Diagnostic Criteria (Spitzer et al. 1978), 46% of those studied had some type of depressive disorder and another 22% had evidence of other depressive features. This same study showed that caregiver wives had a much higher proportion of clinical depression than caregiver husbands—52% versus 21% (Gallagher et al. 1989).

The most frequently cited impact of caregiving is burden, a global concept sometimes linked with stress. Burden conveys the combined sense of oppression, obligation, pervasiveness, and longevity that besets a person in a caregiving situation. Early research found burden to be significantly related to social isolation, particularly by the family, and not to patient symptoms (Zarit et al. 1980). Morycz (1985) found that the desire to institutionalize a care-receiver is strongly related to caregiver strain or burden. The strength of family support, particularly as it facilitates social activity, appears positively related to coping effectiveness (Scott et al. 1986) as well as morale (Gilhooly 1984). Family participation in elder care is so pervasive that one researcher has identified the stress associated with it as developmentally normal (Brody 1985).

A great many studies have tried to establish and delineate the links between patient condition and/or behavior and adverse impact on caregivers. Early work found caregiver well-being to be a more relevant predictor of care outcome (especially institutionalization) than patient variables, suggesting that caregiver characteristics have a greater importance (Colerick and George 1986; George and Gwyther 1986; Gilleard et al. 1982; Zarit et al. 1980). A growing body of work, however, shows that patient variables (condition/behavior) produce adverse effects on caregiver well-being (Niederehe et al. 1983); caregiver gratification (Motenko 1989); quality of care, including patient abuse (Hamilton 1989); and pattern of caregiving, including the type of care provided and the number of family members involved (Birkel and Jones 1989; Brody et al. 1989). Path analytic models have further demonstrated that the combination of patient mental status (especially dementia), troubling symptoms, and troubling behaviors has an adverse impact on caregiver social activity and stress (Deimling and Bass 1986; Noelker 1987). Other work has shown the combined impact of upsetting behaviors and caregiver's perceived competence on the caregiver's stress and sense of reward for the work (Keenan et al. 1989).

Work and caregiving are frequently combined, a trend that, given changing roles of women and patterns of labor force participation, is likely to grow. The combination generally adds to the stress of caregiving. Nearly one-fourth (23%) of the respondents to a large (N = 3,658) employee survey reported assisting an elderly person (Scharlach and Boyd 1989). This added responsibility had several kinds of adverse effects. Caregiving employees were more likely than others to experience interference between jobs and family and to miss work. Approximately 80% of the caregivers reported some kind of strain; caregivers were half again as likely to miss work as noncaregivers (37% versus 23.2%) because of family responsibilities. Other studies have shown that parent care and working produce strain, either by introducing conflict into the work situation or by forcing the caregiving daughter to choose not to work (Brody et al. 1987). Additionally, research shows that working daughters provide as many hours and types of care to impaired mothers as do nonworking daughters; however, the working daughters tend to purchase some of the care rather than provide it directly (Brody and Schoonover 1986).

Caregiver gender relates significantly to coping and the impact of caregiving on the caregiver. Most studies indicate that caregiving is harder on women than on men in terms of burden and depression (Pruchno and Resch 1989), morale (Gilhooly 1984), and initial burden (Zarit et al. 1986). In contrast, Fitting and colleagues (1986) found that the overall experience of caregiving is the same for wives and husbands, but that age related significantly to burden (younger wives and older husbands had higher levels of burden than older wives and younger husbands). Quayhagen and Quayhagen (1988) found that husbands, wives, and children each employed different successful coping mechanisms: all benefited from lower use of fantasy and self-blame; there was a negative association for husbands with physical exercise but a positive one for wives; respite time was positively related to daughters' well-being but negatively so for fathers.

GUIDELINES FOR CLINICAL PRACTICE WITH FAMILY CAREGIVERS

Principles of Care

Clinicians responsible for the care of a chronically ill or impaired elderly person should expect to find a family caregiver involved in the case. In our practice, we expect the caregiver to be an important component of and resource for care and, potentially, a serious casualty of caring. We have distilled the brief review of research, above, into a number of principles that we employ in developing and managing the extended care plan for chronic care patients, as follows:

- *See the dyad.* The caregiving family member and the relationship between him or her and the patient are integral to care continuity. Understanding the caregiver's capabilities, motives, strengths, strains, and relationship to the patient may be as important to care as the patient history and physical examination.
- *Maximize patient functioning.* In addition to promoting a better quality of life for the patient, efforts to treat or reduce excess disability and to use restorative and rehabilitative interventions to raise patient functioning to its highest possible level benefit both patient and caregiver. While minimizing the kind and amount of labor the caregiver is called on to provide, aggressive function-oriented intervention offers a backdrop of control to a situation which, to a caregiver, can seem chaotic and overwhelming.
- *Conserve the caregiver.* The family caregiver holds the care plan in place, often to his or her own detriment. The physician manager must monitor caregiver status (including isolation) and offer whatever therapy, support, and other interventions may be needed to maintain the stability of the caregiving arrangement while protecting the well-being of both the patient and the caregiver.

Issues of Practice

In practice, these principles involve our team in three kinds of broad and ongoing activities. The first of these is caregiver assessment, meant to provide a clear understanding of the family caregiver. The second activity is providing interventions designed to benefit the caregiver. The third activity has to do with the relationship that the clinician and the patient care team both permit and develop with the family caregiver. These issues are discussed in the sections that follow.

Caregiver Assessment

The review of the caregiving literature provides a guide to caregiver assessment. A number of caregiver burden and "hassle" scales are available (Kinney and Stephens 1989; Novak and Guest 1989; Zarit et al. 1980); we sometimes use these as a means of monitoring care-

Table 3-1. Key components of a caregiver assessment

Caregiver characteristics Gender Age Physical condition Live with care receiver Locus of control Other relationships	**Nature of caregiving tasks** What tasks does the caregiver perform How much physical effort How much time at caregiving How long at it Any respite (use and availability)
Relationship with care- **receiver** Stake in caregiving Nature of relationship Strength of relationship	Other caregiving responsibility (i.e., for another family member)
	Skills: Fund of knowledge about patient's disease/condition Actual caregiving skills What learning needs What learning style How skilled at learning Other caregiving experience Coping skills
Socioeconomic status Economic resources Access to services Use of services	
Caregiver work status Working Work-related stress Caregiving stress affecting work	
	Caregiver network What other available members Status of relationships What current involvement by others Potential involvements
Caregiver health and **mental health** Self-reported health status Depression Burden Stress Morale Use of psychotropics, alcohol Presence of other stress	

giver status. Standard depression and anxiety scales can also be useful in detecting problems. However, we attempt to look in detail at the whole person who is providing care in order to develop a complete sense of how this person is functioning as a caregiver; what strains caregiving is putting upon him or her; what forms of help, support, training, and development might prove most useful; what therapies or interventions might best be applied; and in what ways the person might best be incorporated into the patient care team.

Table 3-1 outlines the areas we include in an assessment of a family caregiver. This is not an assessment instrument as such, but we hope a review of the table will sensitize others to the issues we include in our practice approach to caregiver assessment. While the table reflects all of the domains about which we are concerned, its contents are not exhaustive. Any of the points may lead us to probe other areas and in much greater detail. Any assessment area may open the way to a much deeper exploration of some facet of the caregiver which might, in turn, provide us with the clue we need to develop an effective and coherent plan and intervention.

In practice, much of this information is developed over time and by several members of our clinical team. Developing this information is part of the team's overall strategy of forming an alliance with the caregiver. It is also true that, in the process of gathering this information and nurturing the relationship, the team is learning which are the best methods of communicating with the caregiver and which members of the team are best suited for which kinds of communication.

Clinical Interventions

Assessment and a developed relationship and pattern of communication with a caregiver leave us in a position to offer specific and targeted interventions in a timely and appropriate fashion and also to include the caregiver as a part of our care team. In this section we briefly review key interventions that have been used with caregivers and indicate their particular strengths, general indications for their use, and the kinds of outcomes that might be expected from their use. This review is summarized in Table 3-2. The timing and intensity of the use of one or any combination of these interventions are a matter of clinical sensitivity and judgment. The principles governing their use are those cited above concerning the optimization and conservation of the patient-caregiver dyad.

Specialized patient assessments. There are a number of specialized assessments that we consider for any patient with a chronic condition that has major impact on functioning and well-being. The benefits of complete functional assessments have been discussed at length by many authors (American College of Physicians 1988; Katz 1983; Lawton 1971; Williams 1983); similarly, the utility of Geriatric Evaluation Units (GEUs) has been amply documented (Rubenstein et al. 1982, 1984; Solomon et al. 1988). Any suspicion of impaired mental functioning should also prompt a cognitive assessment to determine if an irreversible dementing condition exists.

These assessment strategies represent established techniques and technologies for understanding the complex issues involved in chronic cases and for determining where treatment and rehabilitation poten- tials exist. The assessments benefit the patient directly, but they can also benefit the caregiver. They may lead to interventions that reduce the work of caregiving, e.g., by treating excess disability or by im- proving function. They may also add certainty to a situation and the comfort that everything has been done to learn about the patient's condition and what might be done to cure or contain it. In the ex- treme, assessment can provide the caregiver with the unambiguous knowledge of a terminal prognosis.

In addition to assessments focused on function and pathology, we have begun the practice of conducting values assessments with our patients. Because many of the patients seen in the GRECC clinic are in the early stages of a dementing condition, we promptly conduct values assessments to get direct patient input. A values assessment seeks information about what the person believes about receiving and withholding treatment for himself or herself. This information is useful in three ways. First, it aids us in working with the patient to establish in advance a set of directives for his or her care. Second, it provides us with useful information for working with family care- givers and other family members as the chronic illness runs its course and treatment decisions need to be made. Finally, these values clar- ifications provide family members with information they may find useful in resolving their grief or anger regarding a patient's loss of capacity, institutionalization, and eventual death.

Case management. Another important part of the armamentarium for working with the caregivers of chronically impaired elderly per- sons is case management. Like the GEU, this intervention is well described and documented (Austin 1983). Basically, case manage- ment is the provision of some combination of assessment, care plan- ning, service arrangement and management, and monitoring and periodic reassessment designed to maximize function and to maintain a person in the community. Case management is meant to encompass the kind of practice Eisdorfer and Cohen (1981) describe in speaking of the clinician's role with a dementia patient—the provision of pri- mary care, referral, and information; linkage with legal, financial, and community resources; attention to family well-being; and assis- tance with institutionalization. In our setting, case management also includes specific mechanisms and responsibilities designed to ensure that the patient is connected to the resources he or she needs and that information is reaching the care team in a timely manner to permit plan changes as needed.

We have found that case management services must be differen-

Table 3-2. Caregiver interventions and their characteristics

Interventions	Characteristics	Indications for use	Outcome
Assessments: Functional GEU Cognitive Values	Clarification of patient condition (curable, progressive, terminal) Rule out reversible conditions Treatment plans for excess disability Set advanced directives	Recommended in all cases of chronic illness with major impact	Set clear care goals Maximize patient functioning Minimize work for caregiver Reduce caregiver anxiety
Case management	Assessment Care planning Information Advocacy Service arrangement Monitoring Periodic reassessment	Parsimony Caregiver openness to work with team Caregiver competence Additional informal support Complexities and barriers of the formal system	Ensure patient needs are met Relieve caregiver of undue work Involve other caregivers
Individual counseling	Brief and focused Preventive (for everyone) Situational analysis	Particular conditions—depression, stress, etc. Distress with caregiving	Resolution or amelioration of pathology

Family therapy	Communication problems Perception problems Lack of family resources Ancillary stresses	Source of stress or tension Untapped resources Obvious distress Compliance or other care problems	Reduce caregiver burden and isolation Improve family involvement
Education and training	Specific and tailored Aimed at developing competence	Identified skill or knowledge deficit Change in patient condition	Caregiver skills improved Better care
Support groups	General Aimed at reducing sense of isolation May provide some information	Identified isolation Identified capacity to benefit from group participation	Enhanced socialization and general knowledge
Care team involvement	Care planning Direct care provision In-home case management Clinical observation Treatment initiator	Adjust level of involvement according to caregiver capacity Team membership may extend to other members of the informal network	Better use of caregiver resource Caregiver well-being and esteem

Note. GEU = Geriatric Evaluation Unit.

tially meted out to conform to the caregiver profile that has emerged. We attempt to use the assistance as parsimoniously as possible, so as to build and reinforce caregiver competence and to provide a buffer against the complexities of the formal system when needed.

Individual counseling for caregivers. A number of authors have suggested that individual counseling might be an effective and appropriate intervention with caregivers affected by depression, anxiety, stress, burden, decreased morale, etc. (Rabins 1984; Reifler and Wu 1982). The GRECC psychiatrist regularly sees especially troubled caregivers; his practice with them is typically time-limited and insight-oriented. In addition, we employ a number of individual counseling approaches aimed at helping the caregivers manage the concrete problems presented by the disease and the patient as well as by their own psychological and emotional reactions to the illness. Among the approaches we use are brief problem-focused counseling, supportive therapy, and stress reduction interventions.

Zarit's (1983) brief problem-solving intervention (similar to that described by Herr and Weakland 1983) focuses on helping caregivers to identify the major sources of stress and strain in their lives, to generate and select from alternative solutions, and to follow through in making specific changes. Elsewhere, Zarit and co-workers (1985) have expanded on this counseling strategy, linking the problem identification process with education, problem-solving training, and group support. The primary value of supportive therapy lies in the validation of a caregiver's feelings, the enhancement of self-esteem, and the promotion of self-care (Bonjean 1988). By reviewing the isolation and uncertainty of a caregiving situation with a therapist, a caregiver may be less likely to feel that his or her situation is so unique that others could never understand it and more likely to develop heightened self-esteem. In addition to relaxation training and cognitive behavior approaches designed to interrupt the internal patterns that escalate stress, stress management promotes a sense of mastery or self-efficacy that is linked with superior coping in caregivers (Becker and Coppel 1985; Felton and Revenson 1984; Pearlin et al. 1981).

Family therapy. The link between caregiver burden and family isolation (Zarit et al. 1980) points to the need for the clinician to propose, when appropriate, methods for improving family function by bringing members together to better acknowledge, understand, and organize around the actuality of the chronic illness. Intervention, in this case, can range from taking the practical, intuitive, and brief step of making sure that everyone in the family understands that the patient is really ill and that the caregiver needs help (Gwyther and Blazer 1984; Scott et al. 1986) to initiating an extended course of therapy designed to identify and correct deep-seated problems of family relationships and communication (Kuypers and Trute 1978; Quinn and Keller 1981).

Our major goal in applying family interventions to caregiving situations is to ensure that the family serves as a resource to the caregiver and not as a further source of stress. In general the approaches to family intervention include methods to minimize the discrepancies in perceptions of family members (Blackburn 1988), to clarify role structures and responsibilities (Boss et al. 1988), and to facilitate communication and problem solving (Zarit et al. 1985).

We employ a structured family meeting approach, including all relevant members, in which team members review diagnostic data and treatment recommendations. These meetings help family members to accept the existence and nature of the illness, to develop a consensus about functioning as a supportive team, and to develop a coherent organization of roles and responsibilities to provide this support.

In addition to these one-time family meetings, we also find it useful, in certain circumstances, to initiate a longer, but still brief, course of family therapy. This intervention is focused on strengthening family cohesion and support that have been adversely affected by the disease and caregiving. Brief therapy focused on present day concerns rather than on issues from the past is our preferred approach. We also find it helpful to use mediation techniques as a way to facilitate family decision making about treatment decisions, financial considerations, and institutionalization. Beyond facilitation of problem solving, we use these interventions to help families deal together with the emotional pain and grief associated with the illness.

Education and training.   The notion that family caregivers can benefit from education and training is an intuitively attractive one, particularly to professionals. In practice, the targeted use of educational intervention does seem to be effective. Specific psychoeducational interventions involving cognitive therapy have proved effective in improving morale and lowering depression in family caregivers (Gallagher et al. 1985; Lovett and Gallagher 1988). Cognitive-behavioral approaches in group settings, including those led by peers, have the effect of reducing stress and depression (Gendron et al. 1986; Kahan et al. 1985; Toseland et al. 1989). There is, however, a caveat: While educational interventions have reduced caregiver intolerance of dementia patient behavior (Winogrond et al. 1987) and have mitigated or reduced caregiver burden (Montgomery and Borgatta 1989), it is very important to note that caregivers tend not to use such interventions (see also Oktay and Volland 1990).

We employ two educational strategies in GRECC. First, the team nurse and social worker have organized a sequence of seminars on dementia, community services, legal and financial concerns, and patient management; they are offered monthly and repeated regularly and are open to all caregivers in our clinic. Typically, they are attended by new caregivers. Second, GRECC has produced a series of 21 caregiver education pamphlets (Hepburn 1989) relating to specific issues and problems of caregiving (e.g., working with bureaucracies, dealing with incontinence, selecting a nursing home). The pamphlets are used to supplement counseling and specific teaching interventions. Neither educational intervention is meant or expected to stand alone; both are meant to augment the more direct caregiver teaching and case management activities of the group.

Support groups. Perhaps the best-known form of caregiver intervention is the support group, a strategy that brings together a number of persons whose common bond is caring for a family member. Such groups are led by professionals or trained nonprofessionals knowledgeable about the target condition. Despite the widespread popularity and use of such groups, their impact is limited, though important in its place. Support groups have received early and consistent endorsement from a wide range of professionals (Barnes et al. 1981; George and Gwyther 1983; Safford 1980). These clinicians and others who have conducted more rigorous evaluations of support groups (Clark and Rakowski 1983; Greene and Monahan 1987, 1989; Haley 1989; Haley et al. 1987b; Toseland and Rossiter 1989) have demonstrated that the impact of such groups is modest. They help caregivers to become aware of community resources and to see that they are not alone in their plight, and they help with specific problem-solving. But groups do not have a lasting impact on any of the serious psychological problems that beset caregivers or on their willingness to maintain patients longer in the community. Recognizing that the socialization offered by groups may be somewhat beneficial, we do refer some caregivers to support groups run by the Alzheimer's Association. We do not, however, see support groups as a panacea and, as we have suggested elsewhere, they may be contraindicated for certain caregivers (Hepburn and Wasow 1986).

Care team involvement. Chenoweth and Spencer (1986) have poignantly described the disregard and rejection experienced by family caregivers at the hands of "helping professionals," particularly in medical fields. We have attempted to establish, as the basis of our practice with the chronically ill and their family caregivers, a principle of collegiality or partnership (Maletta and Hepburn 1986; see also Hasselkus 1988 and Imber-Black 1988). It is our perspective that family caregivers are members of the care team, and we expect them to play at least five different roles on the team.

1. They are important in setting the care plan. They know their own capacity for providing care and provide astute and clinically valid assessments of patient condition (see Fischer et al. 1989; Reifler et al. 1981).
2. They are direct care providers, not only in the home but even when patients are institutionalized. They provide care and monitor the care that others provide. (The latter can be disruptive if family members are not included on the team [Bowers 1988].)
3. They can be case managers for the chronically impaired. Their presence affects health care utilization (Fischer and Eustis 1988); and, with guidance, they serve in a gatekeeper role with regard to community services (Caserta et al. 1987). Caregivers can be trained and supervised to play an effective case management role for the chronically impaired (Seltzer et al. 1987; Simmons et al. 1985).
4. They can function on behalf of the clinical team in the home setting. The family gathers clinical observations on which treatment modifications can be based and also plays a significant part in ensuring patient compliance with treatment regimens (Campbell 1987).
5. They sometimes devise and modify treatments, as in the case of adjusting psychotropic medications, with and sometimes without the knowledge of the team. We have observed that many practical home behavior management techniques for dementia patients emanate from successful experimentation by family caregivers.

CONCLUSION

This chapter describes our overall strategy of therapeutic involvement with the caregivers of chronically ill or impaired older persons. In our experience, caregivers are an irreplaceable resource for the care of the chronically ill, but they suffer a plethora of consequences of their work. Our clinical practice with the chronically ill begins with trying to understand the situation of the patient and the caregiver and takes a problem-solving orientation in putting together a plan of care for the dyad. Tactically, we rely on a repertoire of therapeutic interventions, tailoring our approach to the individuals involved and their situation. Most of all, we attempt to involve the caregiver in all aspects of care planning and delivery, and, while monitoring stress and burnout, treat this person as a member of the team as much as possible.

REFERENCES

American College of Physicians, Health and Public Policy Committee: Comprehensive functional assessment for elderly patients. Ann Intern Med 108:70–72, 1988

American Psychiatric Association: Diagnostic and Statistical Manual of Mental Disorders, 3rd Edition, Revised. Washington, DC, American Psychiatric Association, 1987

Austin CD: Case management: options and opportunities. Health Soc Work 8(1):16–30, 1983

Barnes RF, Raskind MA, Scott M, et al: Problems of families caring for Alzheimer patients: use of a support group. J Am Geriatr Soc 19:80–85, 1981

Becker M, Coppel D: Loss of control, self blame and depression: an investigation of spouse caretakers of Alzheimer's disease patients. J Abnorm Psychol 94:169–182, 1985

Birkel RC, Jones CJ: A comparison of the caregiving networks of dependent elderly individuals who are lucid and those who are demented. Gerontologist 29:114–119, 1989

Blackburn J: Chronic health problems of the elderly, in Chronic Illness and Disability, Families in Trouble series Vol 2. Edited by Chillman C, Nunnally E, Cox F. Beverly Hills, CA, Sage, 1988, pp 108–122

Blazer D, Hughes D, George L: The epidemiology of depression in an elderly community population. Gerontologist 27:281–287, 1987

Bonjean M: Psychotherapy for families caring for a mentally impaired elderly member, in Chronic Illness and Disability, Families in Trouble series Volume 2. Edited by Chillman C, Nunnally E, Cox F. Beverly Hills, CA, Sage, 1988, pp 141–155

Boss P, Caron W, Horbal J: Alzheimer's disease and ambiguous loss, in Chronic Illness and Disability, Families in Trouble series Vol 2. Edited by Chillman C, Nunnally E, Cox F. Beverly Hills, CA, Sage, 1988, pp 123–140

Bowers BJ: Family perceptions of care in a nursing home. Gerontologist 28:361–368, 1988

Brody EM: Parent care as a normative family stress. Gerontologist 25:19–29, 1985

Brody EM, Schoonover CB: Patterns of parent-care when adult daughters work and when they do not. Gerontologist 26:372–381, 1986

Brody EM, Lawton MP, Liebowitz B: Senile dementia: public policy and adequate institutional care. Am J Public Health 74:1381–1383, 1984

Brody EM, Kleban MH, Johnson PT, et al: Work status and parent care: a comparison of four groups of women. Gerontologist 27:201–208, 1987

Brody EM, Hoffman C, Kleban MH, et al: Caregiving daughters and their local siblings: perceptions, strains, and interactions. Gerontologist 29:529–538, 1989

Brody SJ, Poulshock SW, Masciocchi CF: The family caring unit: a major consideration in the long-term support system. Gerontologist 18:556–561, 1978

Campbell TL: Families' Impact on Health: A Critical Review and Annotated Bibliography. National Institute of Mental Health series DN, No 6 (DHHS Publ No ADM-87-1461). Washington, DC, U.S. Government Printing Office, 1987

Caserta MS, Lund DA, Wright SD, et al: Caregivers to dementia patients: the utilization of community services. Gerontologist 27:209–214, 1987

Chenoweth B, Spencer B: Dementia: the experience of family caregivers. Gerontologist 26:267–272, 1986

Clark NM, Rakowski W: Family caregivers of older adults: improving helping skills. Gerontologist 23:637–642, 1983

Coe RM, Wolinsky FD, Miller DK, et al: Elderly persons without family support networks and use of health services. Res Aging 7:617–622, 1985

Colerick EJ, George LK: Predictors of institutionalization among caregivers of patients with Alzheimer's disease. J Am Geriatr Soc 34:493–498, 1986

Comptroller General of the United States: Report to Congress: The Well-being of Older People in Cleveland, Ohio. Washington, DC, General Accounting Office, 1977

Comptroller General of the United States: Long-term care for the elderly: issues of need, access, and cost (GAO/HRD-89-4). Washington, DC, General Accounting Office, November 1988

Cross PS, Gurland BJ: The epidemiology of dementing disorders. Report presented to the Office of Technology Assessment, U.S. Congress, 1986

Deimling GT, Bass DM: Symptoms of mental impairment among elderly adults and their effects on family caregivers. J Gerontol 41:778–784, 1986

Eagles M, Craig A, Rawlinson F, et al: The psychological well-being of supporters of the demented elderly. Br J Psychiatry 150:293–298, 1987

Eisdorfer C, Cohen D: Management of the patient and family coping with dementing illness. J Fam Pract 12:831–837, 1981

Felton B, Revenson T: Coping with chronic illness: a study of illness controllability and the influence of coping strategies on psychological adjustment. J Consult Clin Psychol 52:343–353, 1984

Fischer LR, Eustis NW: DRGs and family care for the elderly: a case study. Gerontologist 28:383–398, 1988

Fischer L, Visintainer PF, Schulz R: Reliable assessment of cognitive impairment in dementia patients by family caregivers. Gerontologist 29:333–335, 1989

Fitting M, Rabins P, Lucas MJ, et al: Caregivers for dementia patients: a comparison of husbands and wives. Gerontologist 26:248–252, 1986

Gallagher D, Lovett S, Benedict A, et al: Coping with caregiving: two psychoeducational approaches. Paper presented at annual American Association of Behavioral Therapy meeting, Houston, TX, November 1985

Gallagher D, Rose J, Rivera P, et al: Prevalence of depression in family caregivers. Gerontologist 29:449–456, 1989

Garfinkel SA, Riley GF, Iannacchione VG: High-cost users of medical care. Health Care Financing Review 9:41–52, 1988

Gendron CE, Poitras LR, Engels ML, et al: Skills training with supporters of the demented. J Am Geriatr Soc 34:875–880, 1986

George LK, Gwyther LP: Family caregivers of Alzheimer's patients: correlates of burden and the impact of self-help groups. Paper presented at the annual meeting of the Gerontological Society of America, San Francisco, CA, November 1983

George LK, Gwyther LP: Caregiver well-being: a multidimensional examination of family caregivers of demented adults. Gerontologist 26:253–259, 1986

Gilhooly MLM: The impact of care-giving on care-givers: factors associated with the psychological well-being of people supporting a dementing relative in the community. Br J Med Psychol 57:35–44, 1984

Gilleard CJ, Boyd WD, Watt G: Problems in caring for the elderly mentally infirm at home. Arch Gerontol Geriatr 1:151–158, 1982

Greene VL, Monahan DJ: The effect of a professionally guided caregiver support and education group on institutionalization of care receivers. Gerontologist 27:716–721, 1987

Greene VL, Monahan DJ: The effect of a support and education program on stress and burden among family caregivers to frail elderly persons. Gerontologist 29:472–480, 1989

Gwyther LP, Blazer DG: Family therapy and the dementia patient. Am Fam Physician 29:149–156, 1984

Haley WE: Group intervention for dementia family caregivers: a longitudinal perspective. Gerontologist 29:481–483, 1989

Haley WE, Levine EG, Brown SL, et al: Psychological, social, and health consequences of caring for a relative with senile dementia. J Am Geriatr Soc 35:405–411, 1987a

Haley WE, Brown SL, Levine EG: Experimental evaluation of the effectiveness of group intervention for dementia caregivers. Gerontologist 27:376–382, 1987b

Hamilton G: Prevent elder abuse using a family systems approach. Journal of Gerontological Nursing 15:21–26, 1989

Hasselkus BR: Meaning in family caregiving: perspectives on caregiver/professional relationships. Gerontologist 28:686–691, 1988

Health Care Financing Administration, Office of the Actuary: National health expenditures, 1986–2000. Health Care Financing Review 8:1–36, 1987

Hepburn K: Alzheimer's: a guide for families caring for persons with dementia-related diseases. IB 18-7 and IB 18-7 Suppl 1–20, U.S. Department of Veterans Affairs, August 1989

Hepburn K, Wasow M: Support groups for family caregivers of dementia victims: questions, directions, and future research, in The Elderly and Chronic Mental Illness. Edited by Abramson NS, Quam M, Wason M. San Francisco, CA, Jossey-Bass, 1986, pp 83–92

Herr J, Weakland J: Counseling Elders and Their Families: Practical Techniques for Applied Gerontology. New York, Springer, 1983

Holloway JJ, Thomas JW, Shapiro L: Clinical and sociodemographic risk factors for readmission of Medicare beneficiaries. Health Care Financing Review 10:27–36, 1988

Horowitz A: Family caregiving to the frail elderly, in Annual Review of Gerontology and Geriatrics. Edited by Eisdorfer C. New York, Springer, 1985, pp 194–246

Imber-Black E: The family system and the health care system: making the invisible visible. Journal of Psychotherapy and the Family 4:89–95, 1988

Johnson CL: Dyadic family relations and social support. Gerontologist 23:377–383, 1983

Kahan J, Kemp B, Staples FR, et al: Decreasing the burden in families caring for a relative with a dementing illness. J Am Geriatr Soc 33:664–670, 1985

Katz S: Assessing self-maintenance: activities of daily living, mobility, and instrumental activities of daily living. J Am Geriatr Soc 31:721–727, 1983

Keenan J, Ostwald S, Choi T, et al: Factors that contribute to a caregiver's positive identification with caring for a frail elderly person (abstract). Gerontologist 29 (special issue):83A, 1989

Kinney JM, Stephens MAP: Caregiving hassles scale: assessing the daily hassles of caring for a family member with dementia. Gerontologist 29:328–332, 1989

Kuypers J, Trute B: The older family as the locus of crisis intervention. Family Coordinator 27:405–411, 1978

Lawton MP: The functional assessment of elderly people. J Am Geriatr Soc 19:465–481, 1971

Lovett S, Gallagher D: Psychoeducational interventions for family caregivers: preliminary efficacy data. Behavior Therapy 19:321–330, 1988

Maletta GJ, Hepburn K: Helping families cope with Alzheimer's disease: the physician's role. Geriatrics 41:81–90, 1986

Montgomery RJV, Borgatta EF: The effects of alternative support strategies on family caregiving. Gerontologist 29:457–464, 1989

Mortimer J, Hepburn K, Maletta G: Alzheimer's disease: the intersection of diagnosis, research, and long-term care. Bull NY Acad Med 61:331–342, 1985

Morycz RK: Caregiving strain and the desire to institutionalize family members with Alzheimer's disease. Res Aging 7:329–361, 1985

Motenko AK: The frustrations, gratifications, and well-being of dementia caregivers. Gerontologist 29:166–172, 1989

Niederehe G, Fruge E, Woods AM: Caregiver stress in dementia: clinical outcomes and family considerations. Paper presented at the Annual Scientific Meeting of the Gerontological Society of America, San Francisco, CA, November 1983

Noelker LS: Incontinence in elderly cared for by family. Gerontologist 27:194–200, 1987

Novak M, Guest C: Application of a multidimensional caregiver burden inventory. Gerontologist 29:798–803, 1989

Oktay JS, Volland PJ: Post-hospital program for the frail elderly and their caregivers: a quasi-experimental evaluation. Am J Public Health 80:39–46, 1990

Pearlin L, Lieberman M, Managhan E, et al: The stress process. J Health Soc Behav 22:337–356, 1981

Pruchno RA, Potashnik SL: Caregiving spouses: physical and mental health in perspective. J Am Geriatr Soc 37:697–705, 1989

Pruchno RA, Resch NL: Husbands and wives as caregivers: antecedents of depression and burden. Gerontologist 29:159–165, 1989

Quayhagen MP, Quayhagen M: Alzheimer's stress: coping with the caregiving role. Gerontologist 28:391–396, 1988

Quinn W, Keller J: A family therapy model for preserving independence in older persons: utilization of the family of procreation. American Journal of Family Therapy 9:79–84, 1981

Rabins PV: Management of dementia in the family context. Psychosomatics 25:369–375, 1984

Rabins PV, Mace NL, Lucas MJ: The impact of dementia on the family. JAMA 248:333–335, 1982

Reifler BV, Wu S: Managing families of the demented elderly. J Fam Pract 14:1051–1056, 1982

Reifler BV, Cox GB, Hanley RJ: Problems of mentally ill elderly as perceived by patients, families, and clinicians. Gerontologist 21:165–170, 1981

Rubenstein LZ, Rhee L, Kane RL: The role of geriatric assessment units in caring for the elderly: an analytic review. J Gerontol 37:513–521, 1982

Rubenstein LZ, Josephson KR, Wieland GD, et al: Effectiveness of a geriatric evaluation unit: a randomized clinical trial. N Engl J Med 311:1664–1670, 1984

Safford F: A program for families of the mentally impaired elderly. Gerontologist 20:656–660, 1980

Scharlach AE, Boyd S: Caregiving and employment: results of an employee survey. Gerontologist 29:382–387, 1989

Scott JP, Roberto KA, Hutton JT: Families of Alzheimer's victims: family support to the caregivers. J Am Geriatr Soc 34:348–354, 1986

Seltzer MM, Ivry J, Litchfield LC: Family members as case managers: partnership between the formal and informal support networks. Gerontologist 27:722–728, 1987

Shanas E: Social myth as hypothesis: the case of the family relations of old people. Gerontologist 19:3–9, 1979

Simmons KH, Ivry J, Seltzer MM: Agency-family collaboration. Gerontologist 25:343–346, 1985

Solomon D: Geriatric assessment methods for clinical decision-making. J Am Geriatr Soc 36:342–347, 1988

Spitzer R, Endocott J, Robbins E: Research Diagnostic Criteria: rationale and reliability. Arch Gen Psychiatry 35:773–782, 1978

Stone R, Cafferata GL, Sangl J: Caregivers of the frail elderly: a national profile. Gerontologist 27:616–626, 1987

Toseland RW, Rossiter CM: Group interventions to support family caregivers: a review and analysis. Gerontologist 29:438–448, 1989

Toseland RW, Rossiter CM, Labrecque MS: The effectiveness of peer-led and professionally led groups to support family caregivers. Gerontologist 29:465–471, 1989

U.S. Department of Health and Human Services: Aging America: trends and projections, 1987–88 Edition. Washington, DC, LR 3377(188). D 12198, 1988

Williams TF: Comprehensive functional assessment: an overview. J Am Geriatr Soc 31:637–641, 1983

Winogrond IR, Fisk AA, Kirsling RA, et al: The relationship of caregiver burden and morale to Alzheimer's disease patient function in a therapeutic setting. Gerontologist 27:336–339, 1987

Zarit SH: Interventions with caregivers: do they help and why? Paper presented at the Annual Scientific Meeting of the Gerontological Society of America, San Francisco, CA, November 1983

Zarit SH, Reever KE, Bach-Peterson J: Relatives of the impaired elderly: correlates of feelings of burden. Gerontologist 20:649–655, 1980

Zarit S, Orr N, Zarit N: The Hidden Victims of Alzheimer's Disease: Families Under Stress. New York, New York University Press, 1985

Zarit SH, Todd PA, Zarit JM: Subjective burden of husbands and wives as caregivers: a longitudinal study. Gerontologist 26:260–266, 1986

Chapter Four

PSYCHOTHERAPEUTIC INTERVENTIONS FOR STRESSED FAMILY CAREGIVERS

Dolores Gallagher-Thompson, Ph.D.,
Steven Lovett, Ph.D., and Jon Rose, Ph.D.

The dramatic increase in the number of individuals 65 years and older in the United States has led to a corresponding increase in the number of people who are providing assistance with activities of daily living to older persons suffering from physical or cognitive disabilities (Stone et al. 1987). The majority of older, disabled individuals are being cared for in the home by family members (Johnson and Catalano 1983). Most caregivers who identify themselves as such are women, usually spouses, daughters, or daughters-in-law of the care-receiver (Stone et al. 1987). A recent study suggested that more men may be functioning as caregivers than had been previously thought (Blum et al. 1989). Caregivers were identified based on both self-report and objective criteria of time spent assisting an older individual in daily tasks. It was found that the majority of men objectively identified as caregivers did not see themselves in this role, suggesting that their problems and needs may require separate attention.

Caregiving places enormous demands on the caregiver (George and Gwyther 1986; Stone et al. 1987). Duties may include assisting the care-receiver with personal care activities, supervising all daily activities, managing behavior problems, and managing all financial, legal, and other household duties. Adult children taking care of a disabled parent often face all the demands imposed by their own

---

This work was substantially supported by grants from the National Institute on Aging (AGO-4572) and the National Institute of Mental Health (MH-43407 and MH-40041).

spouses, children, and jobs as well. In addition, there is an emotional toll associated with the decline in health of a loved one, especially in cases of dementia and other cognitive disorders that can drastically alter the care-receiver's basic personality.

The distress experienced by many caregivers is well documented (Daniels and Irwin 1989). Clinical depression was found in 40% to 50% of caregivers who were carefully interviewed by experienced clinicians (Coppel et al. 1985; Gallagher et al. 1989a). Anger appears to be experienced even more commonly (Gallagher et al. 1989b). The negative effects of caregiving have been labeled caregiver burden and numerous studies have both documented its existence and explored its components (Poulshock and Deimling 1984; Vitaliano et al. 1989). Extent of burden appears to be a matter of perception; more is associated not with increasing objectively defined levels of disability, but with how overwhelmed the caregiver feels in his or her particular situation and how well the individual thinks he or she can cope with it (Colerick and George 1986). Recent studies have also suggested that the stress of caregiving may have definite negative consequences on the physical health of the caregiver, ranging from compromised immune system functioning to undetected hypertension and cardiac problems (Kiecolt-Glaser and Glaser 1989; Koin 1989).

TYPES OF SERVICES AVAILABLE

A broad range of different services for caregivers has been described in the literature in several places. (See Gallagher 1985 and an entire special issue of the *Journal of Applied Social Sciences* [Giegel and Blum 1988–89] for reviews.) These services may be categorized into three broad groups.

Respite Programs

The first encompasses various respite-type programs, where the primary aim is to provide the caregiver with "time out" from caregiving responsibilities by providing a safe and supervised place for the impaired elder to be, either several days per week on a regular basis or for an evening, weekend, or longer period (e.g., when family members go on vacation). Respite programs also give direct assistance to the caregiver in terms of specific tasks and activities that need to be done for the impaired elder relative. For example, adult day care and day health programs provide supervised activities and, in the case of day health programs, medical care as well for disabled older adults. Home nursing care, homemaking services, and home sitting services also provide the caregiver with a respite from on-going caregiving and home maintenance duties. The availability of such programs varies from one community to another; generally, consultation from a skilled social worker trained in geriatrics can be very helpful in finding such programs and determining eligibility requirements and the likely extent to which they would be helpful for a particular family.

Support Programs

The second group of services may be called support services. Taken together, their primary aim is to provide the caregiver with infor-mation, skills training, and emotional support to help him or her manage the stress associated with caregiving. The most common ex-ample of this type of service is support groups organized by organi-zations such as the Alzheimer's Disease and Related Disorders Association (ADRDA) and other local and national organizations de-signed to help victims of chronic disease (e.g., Parkinson's disease). These groups sponsor meetings, usually held monthly, are peer-run and frequently provide time for both informational lectures and per-sonal sharing of experiences. Educational workshops sponsored by local hospitals or organizations such as the Visiting Nurses Associ-ation are another example of a support service utilized by many caregivers. Such workshops may focus on information about one or more chronic diseases, legal and financial issues associated with pro-viding care to an older adult, or techniques useful in providing home nursing care (such as transferring, bathing, monitoring medications, etc.).

Psychoeducational Programs

More recently, a number of supportive programs for caregivers have been described that utilize a psychoeducational approach (Gallagher et al. 1989c). This approach expands on the more traditional edu-cational emotional support model by teaching specific psychological skills that can be used by the caregiver to manage stress. Unlike traditional support groups, psychoeducational programs tend to be time-limited and accept only a small number of participants (ap-proximately 10) in each program. There is an agenda for each session and interactive learning is emphasized. Descriptions of three different kinds of psychoeducational programs for family caregivers of the frail elderly that have been developed in our laboratory follow.

The "life satisfaction" class.   This 10-session class was developed originally by Lewinsohn and associates (1984) for use in treating mild depression and related affective distress in younger adults. Content and format were modified by Steinmetz and co-workers (1986) to be more appropriate for the elderly, and subsequent research by Thompson and associates (1983) found that this modality was a very cost-effective intervention for elders in mild to moderate distress who could not or would not seek more formal mental health services. Essentially this class focuses on the relationship between pleasant activities and mood and aims to identify and increase those pleasant activities that are associated with positive mood for each participant. Individual lists of potentially pleasant events and activities are generated and, in the early sessions of the class, participants learn to monitor or "track" their mood level each day, along with recording the frequency of engagement each day in their particular identified pleasant events. After several weeks of observing how mood and events covary, participants are encouraged to discuss barriers that prevent them from an even greater increase in level of positive activities. These might include fear of leaving the frail elderly relative while going out to lunch with a friend; inability to find time in the day to engage in walking, reading, or some other solitary and refreshing activity; and the like. Once identified, class members help each other think through how these obstacles could be reduced or removed, and individual self-change plans are developed and implemented. For example, it may be necessary to do very careful planning so that the frail elder is not left unsupervised while the caregiver engages in a specific pleasant activity, but this is not insurmountable for most caregivers. Or a caregiver may learn that she can find time for herself in certain periods of the day, such as when the frail elder is resting. Others find that by including their relative in more of their activities (depending on the level and types of impairments involved), the relationship improves, leading to identification of more shared pleasant events. Once progress has been made in this area, the class series concludes with discussion of how these skills can be maintained when the class no longer meets regularly. Participants are encouraged to think of future problems with continuing their new routines and to develop ways to remind themselves of our class adage: "Four pleasant events a day keep the blues away."

Mrs. A provides us with an example of how helpful this kind of class can be.

Mrs. A is a 65-year-old wife taking care of her husband, who is disabled from multiple strokes. He needs various kinds of care because of multiple

64

impairments in both physical and cognitive domains. Mrs. A was extremely stressed and depressed when she entered the program and at first was very skeptical that anything as simple as increasing pleasant events in her daily life would be helpful. However, she did agree to try the program for a few weeks before deciding it wasn't for her. She learned that part of her problem was an inability to leave her husband to do things out of the house, for fear he would have another stroke or need some kind of care immediately which she would be unable to provide if she were out enjoying herself. She began with some very small steps: she liked to walk, so the first pleasant activity she put into her program was walking for 10 minutes a day, the maximum time she felt she could safely leave her husband alone in the house. After about a week of this she began (without prodding) to increase her time walking and learned that her husband could not only tolerate her being out of the house for longer periods, but actually enjoyed it himself since it gave him some "breathing room" to begin to identify his own potentially pleasant activities, which he then initiated. Over the 10 weeks of the class a definite increase in pleasant activities developed for both of them with a concomitant improvement in mood and considerably less self-reported stress. On follow-up, Mrs. A indicated that she had "gotten the message" and was becoming more skillful at planning and implementing pleasant activities.

The "problem-solving" class. In contrast, in this class series there is less focus on mood per se and more on learning a model or method for approaching everyday problems that would be more likely to lead to their successful resolution. Since caregivers face a multitude of difficult problems, ranging from daily decisions about the best way of providing care to making long-term financial and legal plans for their impaired relative, this type of class also seemed to hold promise. Psychoeducational programs that teach problem-solving strategies have been shown to be effective interventions for a variety of populations, such as parents learning to cope with teenagers and business managers in supervisory roles. (See D'Zurilla 1986 for a review.) A 10-session program to enhance caregivers' problem-solving skills was developed using material adapted from D'Zurilla (1986). Participants were taught a problem-solving strategy that involved six steps.

1. Achieve a calm state of mind before addressing the problem.
2. Define the problem as specifically as possible.
3. List as many potential solutions to the problem as possible. Do not stop to evaluate them (brainstorming).
4. List the positive and negative points of each potential solution. Identify the "best" solution, i.e., the one most likely to achieve the desired result at the lowest "cost."

5. Carry out the chosen solution.
6. See how well the solution works. If it is not satisfactory, return to step 1 and use the model to identify another potential solution.

The class instructors initially presented the problem-solving model and then facilitated its use during the class sessions as the caregivers described problems they were attempting to solve. The types of problems discussed fell into three broad categories: environmental, personal/emotional, and future problems. Environmental problems included all manner of specific home care, legal, and financial problems. Personal/emotional problems were those that focused primarily on the caregiver's reaction to his or her situation, for example "I am always angry at my husband." Future problems included concerns about who would care for the elder if the caregiver became ill or about the possible need to institutionalize the elder at some future time. Training in problem-solving skills benefited the caregivers by providing them with a framework for addressing the problems they faced and maximizing their chances of finding an effective method of attacking them.

Mrs. B's experience illustrates these benefits.

Mrs. B was a 52-year-old woman who was caring for her 80-year-old mother who lived with Mrs. B and her husband. The mother was physically frail, had significant hearing and vision deficits, and was often confused. Mrs. B initially told the class that her major problem was a continuous feeling of frustration caused by her mother's need for constant supervision. As the problem was clarified, Mrs. B discovered that most of her frustration came from her mother's habit of throwing toilet paper in the waste basket rather than the toilet. All Mrs. B's attempts to reason with her mother on this issue had failed. The class offered a variety of suggestions including removing the waste basket, supervising her visits to the bathroom, arranging for psychological testing, and thinking about the need for a nursing home placement. During the discussion, Mrs. B remembered that when she was growing up, the toilet in the family home never worked properly and was constantly overflowing. Her mother had to constantly unplug it. She thought it was possible that her mother might be reliving this experience and believed that the toilet would overflow if she tried to put toilet paper in it. Another discussion with the class resulted in the idea of putting a brightly colored diaper pail in the bathroom and telling her mother that all toilet paper should be placed in it. This solution would provide a more adequate method of disposing of the toilet paper without trying to convince her mother to use the toilet. The solution was successful and Mrs. B reported that her frustration with her mother had decreased substantially.

The "anger management" class. This class series was developed specifically to help caregivers identify and cope with feelings of anger and frustration, which (besides depression) tend to be extremely common negative emotions in this situation. We found that caregivers tended to be at one extreme or the other on this dimension: some were very easily angered and frequently expressive of their anger, while others were very reserved about this—almost denying such feelings—and often were so unassertive in their dealings with other family members and health care professionals that they allowed themselves to be taken advantage of, with silent resentments building over time. In either case, the extremes were, at times, associated with clear-cut instances of elder abuse or serious neglect. Because of our observation that there was a definite need for a structured intervention to address these issues, we designed this class series. We borrowed from the work of Margaret Chesney and colleagues (1985), who developed anger management classes for stressed business executives, and the work of Feindler and Ecton (1986), who published a manual for the group treatment of hostile adolescents. From these sources plus our own clinical observations about what would be appropriate for this population, we designed a 10-session class that begins with training in how to relax, then teaches a set of cognitive skills, including identification of hostile, defeating self-talk and how to modify it, and concludes with several sessions on assertiveness training. We have found that this particular blend of skills seems to be most effective for anger management.

Participants learn to identify precursors of anger and frustration, such as specific situations that almost always engender this type of response; this is followed by identification of the physiological indices of anger arousal, such as heart pounding, and the introduction of various techniques to stop or slow down the process as it unfolds. In particular, caregivers are asked to pay close attention to their self-talk and to bring it to class meetings for evaluation and modification. They are also asked to log or monitor the frequency of anger-provoking situations and how they are handled. These logs are generally very useful over time as change occurs in either or both dimensions. Similarly, in the assertiveness training portion of the class, caregivers are taught a particular skill (e.g., "broken record" technique, in which a request is politely repeated until a suitable response occurs) and are asked to share their thoughts about it as well. Role-playing is frequently used to give caregivers a chance to practice new behaviors in a safe environment before trying them at home.

Mr. C provides an example of someone who benefited from this type of class.

New Techniques in the Psychotherapy of Older Patients

Mr. C's wife, a moderately severe Alzheimer's disease victim, was a source of great frustration to him, particularly when she continued to repeat questions and statements despite the fact that he answered her and thought that should be the end of it. He found himself becoming extremely angry on an almost daily basis; he attributed this to a belief that she could control her behavior, but was choosing not to in order to "get my goat." He found that a combination of cognitive skills (e.g., reframing her behavior as unintentional, but due to her disease) and behavioral skills (e.g., learning to distract her when the repetitions were particularly frequent) led to diminution of his anger and development of more of a sense of control.

Mrs. D also found these techniques very helpful. She was caring for her sister, who had multiple physical problems but was cognitively intact, yet very demanding. Mrs. D had been extremely passive in her response to her sister, although she described frequent crying in private as an outlet for her frustration. She learned to be more expressive of her feelings and to set limits on what she would and would not do for her sister. Although Mrs. D was acutely uncomfortable at first, she persisted and through modifying her self-talk (i.e., giving herself permission to say "no" at times without feeling guilty) and trying out some new behaviors (learned in class role-playing), she eventually reported definite improvement in mood and well-being.

A more detailed case example follows in which anger was not only experienced, but also expressed in ways that were excessive and amounted to physical abuse. This caregiver was first treated in the anger management class where he made definite improvement in that the abusive episodes were much less frequent after his class participation. However, he felt, and we agreed, that more intensive individual therapy was needed, so he was given 16 sessions of cognitive-behavioral therapy in Project Assist. (That project will be described in more detail below.)

Mr. E was a 60-year-old caregiver of a rather frail younger brother (Robert) who had been diagnosed with multi-infarct dementia (MID). Robert had been an alcoholic earlier in life and was the type of person who settled disagreements with verbal and/or physical abuse. Mr. E and his brother had begun sharing a household following the deaths of both their wives about 5 years before. Shortly thereafter, Robert had a series of strokes, the last of which resulted in substantial cognitive and physical impairment. Mr. E felt guilty about doing anything other than keeping his brother in the home with him, although Robert's disabilities were very distressing to him and Robert's increasing hostility and angry verbal outbursts were hard to handle. At the same time, Mr. E was developing a romantic interest and resented not being able to follow through with that as he pleased; instead he felt quite inhibited by his brother's

68

presence in his home. The situation gradually worsened to the point where the two brothers were given to frequent angry outbursts leading, at times, to Mr. E hitting Robert on the shoulder or upper arm. Afterwards he would feel extremely guilty about this and concerned that he might lose control during one of these episodes and actually hurt his brother or somehow cause another stroke.

When Mr. E joined the anger management class, he seemed ready to learn some of the methods for greater self-control in frustrating situations. He particularly benefited from two interventions: first, reading and learning more about MID and its variable, step-wise course; and second, learning to challenge his belief that his brother was not as mentally disabled as he appeared, but was merely intentionally acting out his old alcoholic pattern of trying to get others to take care of him while he was irresponsible. By carrying out behavioral experiments in the home (e.g., trying to think of ways for his brother to be more independent), he was able to garner concrete evidence of the very real limitations that were present. Mr. E also learned to focus more on the positives in their relationship, such as the fact that they met some of each other's emotional needs by living together and could still share some very pleasant activities such as fishing and watching ballgames on television. However, after the 10 sessions of the class had concluded, it was evident that Mr. E was still troubled by his less frequent angry outbursts and by his fear that he would unintentionally harm his brother. Individual cognitive-behavioral therapy was then initiated through the "Assist" program. During the 16 sessions, Mr. E learned ways to curtail his anger even further (e.g., by setting limits on when he would be home and how he would handle the situation with his new female companion) and by honestly assessing the pros and cons of continuing to share a home with his brother. Other family members (e.g., a daughter and several nieces who lived locally) were brought into the picture and even attended some of the therapy sessions along with the client, in order to develop more of a support network for both brothers. Finally, over time, Mr. E was able to accept the severity of his brother's impairments and stop viewing his behavior as intentional. When that occurred, the abusive verbal and physical behavior stopped altogether. By the time of the 2-month follow-up, it was evident that Mr. E was able to maintain his improved emotional state through the continued use of more realistic and adaptive self-talk and through more reliance on the available social support network to help balance out the caregiving load.

Individual Counseling and Psychotherapy

An additional category of services includes various approaches for individual counseling and/or psychotherapy with family caregivers. It is necessary to have these kinds of services available in one's armamentarium because there are a number of caregivers who suffer from clinical depression, alcohol abuse, severe anxiety, and the like—and even some who commit elder abuse or neglect—who need more intensive service. In our experience, both cognitive/behavioral approaches and time-limited psychodynamic psychotherapy can be very effective with caregivers in more serious psychological distress who need individual assistance. However, it is not always easy to engage caregivers in individual psychotherapeutic treatment. For many, it is a sign of weakness or defeat; others focus so strongly on the needs of their frail elderly relative that they virtually ignore their own warning signs and do not seek professional help until the problem is severe enough to interfere with their daily lives.

Project Assist is a federally funded research project designed to study the effectiveness of two forms of brief psychotherapy for treating acute psychological distress associated with caring for a chronically ill relative at home. It was developed because a number of caregivers that we evaluated for the class programs were too emotionally distressed to be appropriately treated in a class format and/or asked for individual counseling time. Although we did not envision the need for such a program at first, we soon were impressed with the demand for service. However, rather than simply provide services, we decided to investigate whether or not one type of therapy would be more effective than the other, based on such individual-difference variables as length of time as a caregiver and whether or not the person being cared for was cognitively impaired. To date we have treated about 75 caregivers in this clinical research program. Although the study is still in progress and definitive results will not be available until late 1991, preliminary data indicate that results will be consistent with most psychotherapy outcome studies. By this we mean that approximately two-thirds of those who engaged in either treatment (i.e., remained after three sessions) were either in full remission or substantially improved by the end of therapy, and most were able to maintain their gains for about one year following termination. The two treatments utilized were cognitive-behavioral therapy, as outlined in Beck et al. (1979) and Lewinsohn et al. (1986), and time-limited psychodynamic therapy, as described in Mann (1973). Both treatments consisted of approximately 20 individual sessions of about an hour's duration each, conducted by a doctoral-level therapist and supervised by a more senior therapist. The initial eight sessions were spaced twice per week, and the remaining 12 were weekly, although patients' schedules and holidays sometimes interrupted this schedule.

Cognitive-Behavioral Therapy

Cognitive-behavioral therapy proposes that mental disorders, particularly depression, can be alleviated by teaching clients new skills for identifying maladaptive thoughts, forming adaptive cognitions, and altering maladaptive behavioral patterns. While techniques are initially learned and rehearsed in the therapy sessions, graded in vivo experience applying the techniques (called "homework") is considered to be a critical ingredient of change. Detailed descriptions of this modality can be found in the references cited above, and in Chapter 1.

Of particular interest here is the identification of maladaptive thought patterns that are common in family caregivers and how to counteract the negative effects of these thoughts. Dichotomous thinking (variously labeled "all or nothing" or "black and white") is one of the most common thought distortions of all depressed people. Among caregivers, there are several common manifestations of this theme. "This person is no longer my husband" is one example. "I got angry at my mother for something she frequently does, so I am a bad person for not being more understanding" is another variant. "Mind-reading" is another habit that often leads to distress. Many people assume they know what others are thinking or feeling without bothering to verify their intuition. This can lead to inaccurate attributions of intentionality when care-receivers behave in a way that is upsetting to the caregiver. It can also lead to misguided empathy which results in unnecessary caregiver distress. For example, upon observing a demented spouse tearing paper napkins, a caregiver may imagine how frustrating it would be if he or she couldn't think of anything better to do. Actually, many demented individuals enjoy this activity. Since most caregivers knew their charges well prior to the disability, it is often difficult for them to accept that nonlinguistic cues may no longer carry the same meaning as before. This can make "mind-reading" errors difficult for the caregiver to identify. Another serious problem often brought to therapy sessions is the insistence that the well-being of caregiver and patient are rigidly interdependent. Thus, when a caregiver is asked "How are you feeling?" he or she will often describe the frail elder's mood or health. Similarly, many caregivers unfairly blame themselves if the person they care for is unhappy. Techniques such as the Dysfunctional Thought Record can be used to monitor the occurrence of these cognitive distortions and to learn how to generate more adaptive alternative explanations and perceptions. It is also common to include behavioral skills, such as role playing and relaxation training, in the therapy program in order to help the caregiver integrate changes more fully into his or her daily life.

Time-Limited Psychodynamic Therapy

In contrast to cognitive and behavioral skill training is the model of time-limited psychodynamic therapy developed by Mann (1973) and used as the basis for the dynamic therapy provided in Project Assist. This modality is designed to utilize the existential experience of time in the therapeutic relationship and is based on "the recurring life crisis of separation-individuation" as described by Mahler et al. (1975, p. 24). This theoretical underpinning proved to be quite fortuitous because we soon noted that many caregivers seen in Project Assist appeared to be struggling with this very developmental issue. For example, many of the patients seen for individual psychotherapy in the psychodynamic modality reported frequent difficulty separating their own thoughts, feelings, identity, and sense of well-being from those of the care-receiver. Yet this process appears necessary for the individuation and mental health of caregivers (Rose 1989).

Psychologically "healthy" caregivers are expected to recognize accurately the presence or absence of conflict between people and to imagine solutions to meet the most important needs of all concerned, without severing the relationship. Caregivers with acute psychopathology are often inaccurate in the perception of conflict and imagine resolutions involving significant and unrewarded sacrifice of one party or severing of the relationship (Rose 1989). However, in brief psychodynamic therapy, there is an opportunity to understand past conflicts in separation-individuation through their reenactment in the therapeutic relationship. Relatives of persons with deteriorating illness experience a succession of losses. The sense of loss may be acute regardless of prior satisfaction with the relationship. This is because the frail relative was familiar and fulfilled important (whether pleasant or unpleasant) psychological and social functions that beg replacement (Rose and DelMaestro 1988).

Caregivers' ability to grieve and individuate is often hampered by the incompleteness of the separation—the frail elder is still present, but his or her psychological and/or social function to the caregiver is gone. In this process, the familiar "object" of one's affection is transformed into the unfamiliar. Caregivers appear to struggle between a desire to increase psychological distance from their frail relative and wanting to restore their perception of the person who was familiar and important. Unlike young children who can be reassured of a continuing relationship with the parent as they become more autonomous, caregivers face the impending death of their loved one as they become more individuated, and often experience guilt about their need to separate, experiencing survivorship as abandonment.

The next case example illustrates some of the key active ingredients of therapy in Project Assist.

> Mrs. F was a 40-year-old moderately clinically depressed married woman who wanted to "feel good again." She was a caregiver for her 85-year-old mother who suffered from severe rheumatoid arthritis and very poor hearing. The mother had, for years, lived with her son in another state for a portion of the year and with Mrs. F for the remainder of the year. The caregiver's target complaints on entering therapy included the following: 1) feeling caught between her mother and her family; 2) feeling unappreciated by her mother; and 3) communication problems with her brother and his wife about their mother's care, particularly with regard to future plans and living arrangements.

The precipitant for Mrs. F's seeking help was that when her mother moved back in with her most recently, Mrs. F became clinically depressed as a result. The patient stated that their communication had deteriorated and many of their interactions ended up with both of them crying and feeling upset and frustrated. In addition, there was much stress and conflict in Mrs. F's family over her mother's presence in the home this time, possibly because she was much less functional than in previous years. Mrs. F's main goal was to improve communication with her mother and her family both in terms of effectiveness and pleasantness. Mrs. F had no previous treatment for depression, though she did acknowledge communication problems with her mother since she was a child (i.e., feeling dominated). She reported no other emotional problems prior to becoming a caregiver. Mrs. F lived in her own home with her husband of 20 years and two teenaged children. The rest of her relatives, including her brother, lived in the Midwest. She had 3 years of college and had worked as a secretary but could not continue when this depression developed. This put an extra hardship on the family, who had grown accustomed to her additional income.

Mrs. F received 21 sessions of individual cognitive-behavioral therapy addressing her dysfunctional thinking as well as building communication and assertiveness skills. The dysfunctional thinking occurred particularly around conflicts with the mother and brother and around her brother's decision to place their mother in a nursing home when she returned to his home later in the year.

Using Dysfunctional Thought Records, Mrs. F listed her distorted thoughts, negative feelings, and more adaptive ways of thinking. Some examples of her negative thoughts included: "I am an uncaring, bad person for allowing my mother to be placed in a nursing home"; "I should care for my mother all of the time, even if it gets in the way of my own needs and those of my family"; "My brother is a jerk—he is doing everything the wrong way"; and "All nursing homes are horrible places." Negative feelings that arose included anger, frustration, guilt, and anxiety. Some of the main cognitive distortions used by Mrs. F were identified as "all or nothing thinking," "jumping to conclusions," and "should statements." By evaluating these cognitive distortions and coming up with more adaptive perspectives, such as "I need to balance my mother's needs with my own needs and my family's needs" and "My brother is doing certain things well in caring for my mother and other things less well," her level of stress was reduced.

One way of helping Mrs. F deal with her dysfunctional thinking was to teach her communication and assertiveness skills so she could express herself more directly and elicit information more directly from others. By being more direct, she was less likely to make assumptions and try to read other's minds or expect them to read her mind. These skills were presented and then practiced through role-playing of a problematic interaction from the past or an anticipated difficult situation that she wanted to prepare for. Role-playing was used to help her improve communication not only with her mother, but also with her brother and sister-in-law, her mother-in-law, her husband, and her children. Improved communication and assertiveness skills seemed to generalize to many areas of her life.

At the end of treatment, Mrs. F and her therapist collaborated on developing the following "survival guide" that listed the coping skills she had acquired over the course of therapy and could use in the future to prevent relapse.

Survival guide

To use with mother:
1. Make sure I have her attention (be sure her hearing aid is in and say directly: "I need to talk to you about something important").
2. Remember I have gotten positive results when I have been persistent.
3. I know it is stressful to push topics with her, but usually in the long run getting it out in the open can reduce stress.

In interactions with own family:

1. Try to ask family members directly for their reasons for suggesting something and try not to assume the "real" reason or intention might be different from what they say.
2. Give feedback to family members about their effect on me because they may not realize their impact.

In interactions with brother and sister-in-law:

1. When I want to call them, plan to do so when I have plenty of time (may have to call several times in order to reach brother).
2. Set an agenda of what I want to cover in the conversation and how I want to broach the subjects.
3. Consider nurturing relationship with brother and sister-in-law by not always calling about mother or on business.

Regarding future plans for mother:

1. Evaluate mother's care needs: Where might she get the best care: In our home? With a home health aide? In a local nursing home until her strength is built up?
2. Evaluate my own family's needs: How can her needs and our needs be worked out?
3. What does mother really want? What are her preferences?

At the end of treatment, Mrs. F rated all of her initial target complaints as greatly eased. She was no longer clinically depressed and she clearly was functioning in more adaptive ways at home. When she was seen for follow-up 3 months later, it was evident to the interviewer that Mrs. F was maintaining her gains. She and her brother and mother had worked collaboratively on selecting a residential care setting that would be satisfactory to all parties, and although definite plans had not yet been finalized, they clearly were in the offing. Considering the extent of her initial distress, Mrs. F can be regarded as a client for whom Project Assist was very helpful.

It should be noted at this point that this client would most likely have had an equally favorable outcome had she received time-limited psychodynamic therapy, since issues of separation and individuation were clearly central to her distress. Clinically, we have observed that several other clients with similar issues were very effectively treated with dynamic therapy, leading us to conclude that for many caregivers with reactive depressions, either treatment is likely to be effective depending on the expertise of the therapist.

In summary, our clinical experience with these two very different types of therapy—cognitive-behavioral therapy and time-limited psychodynamic therapy—strongly suggests that they are both of value to caregivers in distress. Our research data, while preliminary at this point, support this conclusion. Although we do not know what mechanisms are responsible for change in each type of treatment, we do know that, given the opportunity, caregivers will enthusiastically participate in brief therapies that seem to address their specific concerns and issues.

SUMMARY

We hope that this chapter has given the reader a good idea of the types of psychoeducational and psychotherapeutic interventions that we have been using successfully and that we recommend to other mental health professionals who are just beginning to work with caregivers. As noted earlier in this chapter, many caregivers attend support groups regularly and, for some, this type of intervention may be sufficient to meet their needs. Since caregivers tend to be very good copers in general (Horowitz 1985), we recommend being careful not to overly "pathologize" their distress. Rather, in our opinion, the goal of treatment is to help them overcome whatever blocks are reducing their sense of self-efficacy in the situation. We believe that the various time-limited therapies are very appropriate for this purpose, while still acknowledging that for some caregivers more may be needed (e.g., psychotropic medication or long-term therapy). However, in our experience, this would be a small group, distinguished primarily by their own history of mental illness or serious personality disorder. The majority of caregivers we and our colleagues have treated benefited from the types of interventions described here.

It seems to us that a major challenge for the future in the treatment of family caregivers involves being able to identify at intake who may be most likely to benefit from which type of treatment. More information is needed about the characteristics of caregivers most likely to benefit from one of the structured class approaches versus those who need and can benefit from the more intensive individual psychotherapeutic work (irrespective of preferred modality). Similarly, there may be some caregivers who will be helped more by a cognitive-behavioral approach, while others resonate much more to the psychodynamic orientation. The identification of factors associated with success in each of these modalities is research yet to be done.

A related topic that needs more study is the interplay among various types of services. Earlier it was noted that respite-type services and self-help groups were two kinds of interventions that many caregivers sought and used heavily. But we do not know if these services have some kind of additive or multiplicative function—the more you participate the better you feel—or if they are sufficiently unique that caregivers should be encouraged to use one (or two, at most) at a time. Given economic constraints and fewer resources in the years ahead, these questions require serious attention in the not too distant future.

REFERENCES

Beck AT, Rush AJ, Shaw BF, et al: Cognitive Therapy of Depression. New York, Guilford Press, 1979

Biegel DE, Blum A (eds): Special issue: aging and family caregivers. J Applied Soc Sci 13:1–250, 1988–89

Blum M, Kelley M, Gatz M: Empirically defined caregivers versus self-defined caregivers for aging parents. Paper presented at the annual meeting of the Gerontological Society of America, Minneapolis, MN, November 1989

Chesney M: Anger and hostility: future implications for behavioral medicine, in Anger and Hostility in Cardiovascular and Behavioral Disorders. Edited by Chesney MA, Rosenman RH. Washington, DC, Hemisphere, 1985, pp 277–290

Colerick EJ, George LK: Predictors of institutionalization among caregivers of patients with Alzheimer's disease. J Am Geriatr Soc 34:493–498, 1986

Coppel DB, Burton D, Becker J, et al: Relationships of cognitions associated with coping reactions to depression in spousal caregivers of Alzheimer's disease patients. Cognitive Therapy and Research 9:253–266, 1985

Daniels M, Irwin M: Caregiver stress and well-being, in Alzheimer's Disease Treatment and Family Stress (DHHS Publ No 89-1569). Edited by Light E, Lebowitz B. Washington, DC, U.S. Government Printing Office, 1989, pp 292–309

D'Zurilla TJ: Problem-solving Therapy. New York, Springer, 1986

Feindler EL, Ecton RB: Adolescent Anger Control: Cognitive-Behavioral Techniques. New York, Pergamon Press, 1986

Gallagher D: Intervention strategies to assist caregivers of frail elders: current research status and future research directions, in Annual Review of Gerontology and Geriatrics, Vol 5. Edited by Lawton MP, Maddox G. New York, Springer, 1985, pp 249–282

Gallagher D, Rose J, Rivera P, et al: Prevalence of depression in family caregivers. Gerontologist 29:449–456, 1989a

Gallagher D, Wrabetz A, Lovett S, et al: Depression and other negative affects in family caregivers, in Alzheimer's Disease Treatment and Family Stress (DHHS Publ No 89-1569). Edited by Light E, Lebowitz B. Washington, DC, U.S. Government Printing Office, 1989b, pp 218–244

Gallagher D, Lovett S, Zeiss A: Interventions with caregivers of frail elderly persons, in Aging and Health Care: Social Science and Policy Perspectives. Edited by Ory M, Bond K. London, Routledge Press, 1989c, pp 167–190

George LK, Gwyther L: Caregiver well-being: a multidimensional examination of family caregivers of demented adults. Gerontologist 26:253–259, 1986

Horowitz A: Family caregiving to the frail elderly, in Annual Review of Gerontology and Geriatrics, Vol 5. Edited by Lawton MP, Maddox G. New York, Springer, 1985, pp 194–246

Johnson CL, Catalano D: A longitudinal study of family supports to the impaired elderly. Gerontologist 23:612–618, 1983

Kiecolt-Glaser JK, Glaser R: Caregiving, mental health, and immune function, in Alzheimer's Disease Treatment and Family Stress (DHHS Publ No 89-1569). Edited by Light E, Lebowitz B. Washington, DC, U.S. Government Printing Office, 1989, pp 245–266

Koin D: The effects of caregiver stress on physical health status, in Alzheimer's Disease Treatment and Family Stress (DHHS Publ No 89-1569). Edited by Light E, Lebowitz B. Washington, DC, U.S. Government Printing Office, 1989, pp 310–320

Lewinsohn PM, Antonuccio DO, Steinmetz JL, et al: The Coping With Depression Course: A Psychoeducational Intervention for Unipolar Depression. Eugene, OR, Castalia, 1984

Lewinsohn PM, Munoz R, Youngren MA, et al: Control Your Depression, Revised Edition. Englewood Cliffs, NJ, Prentice-Hall, 1986

Mahler MS, Pine F, Bergman A: The Psychological Birth of the Infant: Symbiosis and Individuation. New York, Basic Books, 1975

Mann J: Time-Limited Psychotherapy. Cambridge, MA, Harvard University Press, 1973

Poulshock SW, Deimling GT: Families caring for elders in residence: issues in the measurement of burden. J Gerontol 39:230–239, 1984

Rose J: The Role of Separation-Individuation in Determining Wives' Ability to Care for Disabled Husbands. Doctoral dissertation, Northwestern University. Chicago, IL, 1989

Rose J, DelMaestro S: Separation-individuation conflict as a model for understanding caregiver distress. Paper presented at the annual meeting of the Gerontological Society of America, Minneapolis, MN, November 1989

Steinmetz J, Zeiss AM, Thompson LW: The life satisfaction course: an intervention for the elderly, in The Prevention of Depression: Research Foundations. Edited by Munoz R. Washington, DC, Hemisphere, 1986

Stone R, Cafferata GL, Sangl J: Caregivers of the elderly: a national profile. Gerontologist 27:616–631, 1987

Thompson LW, Gallagher D, Nies G, et al: Evaluation of the effectiveness of professionals and nonprofessionals as instructors of "Coping with Depression" classes for elders. Gerontologist 23:390–396, 1983

Vitaliano PP, Mauro RD, Ochs H, et al: A model of burden of caregivers of DAT patients, in Alzheimer's Disease Treatment and Family Stress (DHHS Publ No 89-1569). Edited by Light E, Lebowitz B. Washington, DC, U.S. Government Printing Office, 1989, pp 267–291

Chapter Five

SOCIAL NETWORK THERAPY WITH INNER-CITY ELDERLY

Carl I. Cohen, M.D.

In its most basic form a social network can be defined as a scattering of points connected by lines. The points are persons and the lines are social relations. Diagrammatically, the social network is analogous to a communication circuit: it indicates that certain persons are in touch with each other (Boissevain 1974). The definition has generally been broadened to include the notions that the characteristics of the linkages may be used to interpret the social behavior of the persons involved (Mitchell 1969), to help an individual maintain his or her social identity, and to provide for the exchange of emotional support, material aid, and information (Walker et al. 1977). The latter concept of a network as a support system is particularly relevant to clinicians and service providers, although it should be underscored that network linkages can be deleterious as well as beneficial.

Empirical findings and methodological advances over the past two decades, which are discussed below, make this a propitious time to consider the clinical relevance of social network interventions for use with the elderly, particularly those residing in the inner-city. The idea of personal connections is so fundamental that it has been taken for granted, and only in the past few years has it been studied systematically (Hammer et al. 1976). Over the past

Partial support for this work was provided by the Ittleson, Van Amerigen, and New York foundations. I thank Carole Lefkowitz, Jay Sokolovsky, Arlene Adler, and Joan Mintz for their assistance.

79

three decades, commencing with the studies by Barnes (1954) of a Norwegian parish and Bott (1957) of a London neighborhood, the concept of "social network" has evolved from a metaphor into a precisely defined analytic concept. By the late 1970s, network analysis began to be applied to geriatric research and practice (Cohen and Sokolovsky 1979; Pilisik and Minkler 1980; Snow and Gordon 1980).

During the 1960s, as clinicians left their desks and moved into the community, they began to recognize the role that social networks played in the daily lives of their clients. Working among the elderly and poor, clinicians realized that individual-oriented therapy could not completely address the problems confronting their clients. Experimental treatment strategies within the social network system began to emerge. Empirical research also indicated that elderly persons residing in the community have viable informal support systems composed primarily of geographically close family and friends (Gottlieb 1983). Even the most marginal elderly populations were found to have active social supports. For example, homeless older men in New York City had 8.5 network contacts that they saw on an average of 3.6 times per week. There were no persons without any linkages and only 12% had two or fewer social ties (Cohen and Sokolovsky 1989).

Numerous studies have found that greater levels of social support have a direct positive influence on health, regardless of the degree of stress (Gottlieb 1983). There is also substantial evidence to support a stress-buffering effect for social networks in many clinical conditions, i.e., social support can moderate the effects of increased stress on health (Gottlieb 1983). Moreover, in healthy older adults, strong social supports appear to favorably influence various physiological measures such as immune function and cholesterol levels (Thomas et al. 1985).

A final source of influence on social network intervention has arisen from what consumers and the community perceive as major gaps in the delivery system. From the consumer side, there has been a sense that professional care is too impersonal, tends to downplay the patient's role in effecting change, and generally ignores the therapeutic role of close family and friends. Consequently, many people have begun to develop and participate in various mutual aid groups (Gottlieb 1981). In addition, the inconsistency of governmental funding in recent years has compelled service providers in the community to explore the value of natural support networks in helping to meet at least some of their clients' needs.

CHARTING SOCIAL NETWORKS:
THE NETWORK ANALYSIS PROFILE

In our work, we endeavored to create an instrument—the Network Analysis Profile (NAP)—that would combine the best features of sociological and anthropological network methods (Sokolovsky and Cohen 1981). That is, in the former mode it would permit us to chart large numbers of people with respect to quantitative aspects of networks (e.g., size, density), and in the latter it would enable us to elicit information about qualitative network features (e.g., content of exchanges, subjective feelings). The NAP yields information in three sectors of interaction: non-kin (e.g., friends, acquaintances), kin, and formal (e.g., social workers, physicians, clergy). In charting a network, the interviewer usually begins with the non-kin sector and asks the respondent to name as many persons as he or she has seen or heard from in a particular sector in the past 3 months. He or she may add other names of people seen or heard from in the past year if they are considered important. The respondent is then asked about persons in the next sector. For persons with cognitive deficits, relatives or significant collaterals can help to chart the network.

For each person in the network, the respondent is asked questions aimed at determining various interactional and structural features of the network. Interactional characteristics include the frequency and duration of the interaction, the direction and flow of the aid, the levels of intimacy and of subjective importance, and an analysis of transactional content. With respect to the latter, "uniplex" relations in which linkages deal with only one type of content, e.g., food aid, medical assistance, loans, are differentiated from "multiplex" relationships that contain more than one content. Structural characteristics include size, density, and clustering. Density is defined as the ratio of actual to potential links in a network and clustering refers to compartments of networks that have a relatively high density.

CLINICAL APPROACHES

The key feature of a network approach is that the therapist employs the older person's social network system to deal with problems. Clients may present with emotional as well as instrumental (e.g., housing, medical aid, shopping) needs. Two distinct network approaches have emerged in work with older persons (Biegel et al. 1984). One approach, developed by John Garrison (Garrison 1974; Garrison and

Howe 1976), involves the actual convening of members of the individual network into a "network session" in which a treatment plan is developed and sponsored by network members themselves. A second approach, developed by our group (Cohen and Sokolovsky 1979, 1981), involves the clinician's utilizing the network on the client's behalf, usually by working with network members to elicit their involvement in the client's treatment.

Biegel (1984) points out that the network session approach is more highly specialized and requires substantial training. The second approach involves less change from the usual mode of clinical practice. Even though it may involve a shift from a psychodynamic to a more systems-oriented practice, it is generally more easily accepted by staff members (Biegel 1984). As a practical matter, the network session has been used almost exclusively with older persons living in intact families. It may be especially well-suited for those lower income elderly who, despite having smaller networks than their middle-class counterparts, have networks concentrated on family members (Antonucci 1985). Lack of experience notwithstanding, there is no reason why this technique cannot be employed with older persons living alone.

Network Session Approach

Garrison's network approach is based on the assumption "that the solution to a variety of human dilemmas lies within the expectations and collective resources of an individual's social network" (Garrison and Howe 1976, p. 330). The goals of the intervention should be to modify the emotional influence that the network has on the client, with the aim of promoting active reality-based coping with problems, and to articulate which instrumental resources (professional caregivers, community agencies, and other significant supports) are needed.

The vehicle for involving the client's social network in the treatment process is the network session. The network session is usually held in the client's home and involves convening relevant members of his or her social network, including family, friends, agency staff, etc. Garrison and Howe (1976) identify four criteria necessary to assess whether social network intervention is appropriate: 1) There must be emotional or instrumental resources in the client's social environment that can be beneficial; 2) caregivers must be open to a network approach; 3) the client must be willing to convene the important people in his or her life; 4) there should be no contraindication to using the network approach (e.g., client is too paranoid or cannot control physical impulses).

Once the therapist obtains the client's permission to convene a network session, the first step is to list those members who play a significant role in the client's life. Although Garrison specifies no charting method, the Network Analysis Profile is suitable for such an exercise. A time for the network session is set and the clinician or client telephones each person on the list to invite them to the meeting. The meeting is described to the participants as a problem-solving session to help the client find a solution to his or her current difficulties. Garrison notes that he intentionally omits the word "therapy" to avoid stimulating any unnecessary anxiety.

Garrison and Howe (1976) described five essential components of the Network Session:

1. Inventory the elements of the situation and define specific problem(s) (e.g., client not going outside, client pacing).
2. List alternative courses of action (e.g., home care, medication, hospitalization).
3. List pros and cons for each alternative.
4. Decide on an alternative and test it, defining specific criteria for improvement (e.g., client will go out for 15 minutes each day).
5. Evaluate outcome and start over if necessary (e.g., a second session is scheduled to obtain feedback).

Reminiscing is encouraged during sessions, and photograph albums and memorabilia may receive lengthy attention. Garrison and Howe (1976) argue that the revival of memories is important to clarify the identity of the older client.

Network Sessions generally include between 5 and 30 persons and last from 1 to 3 hours. Ordinarily, the client will participate in two or three sessions spaced from 2 to 8 weeks apart.

The Individual-Centered Approach

During our clinical and research work with older persons living in single-room occupancy hotels in midtown Manhattan, we became increasingly cognizant of the important role that the social support system played in maintaining these persons in the community. We began to experiment with a variety of social network techniques. In the following section, I describe the clinical uses and principal network techniques that have evolved from our work with inner-city elderly populations.

Use at the service agency level. Network analysis can be particularly valuable in sensitizing service personnel to the notion that their clients have active personal networks and are not complete "isolates"; nor are they incapable of engaging in affective interactions. As an illustration, in mapping the networks of 161 elderly single-room occupancy residents, the mean number of contacts was found to be 7.8, with more than four-fifths of these links involving multiplex relations (Cohen et al. 1985). More significant, one-third of all links involved the exchange of sustenance items such as food, money, or medical assistance. Two-thirds of the residents reported at least one intimate relationship. Three-fourths of all relationships occurred outside the hotel, and as others have reported (Bengston 1979; Cantor 1975), family ties of the urban aged are far from totally severed. For these hotel elderly, one-third of all relationships involved links to kin.

Although it is important to overcome worker biases concerning single-room occupancy "isolation," it is equally crucial to alert them to the diversity in network magnitude and intensity. Networks ranged in size from 0 to 26, and although 4 persons had no multiplex relationships, 15 individuals had networks of 15 or more multiplex relationships.

Network analysis can also be used to help agency staff see individual behavior in the context of systems. The focus of community treatment has been chiefly on the individual in need of help. Although community practice has expanded to include a multidisciplinary approach, new problems continue to be viewed as an individual matter, with little emphasis placed on the total set of systems surrounding the person (Biegel et al. 1984). Network analysis is a "systems" theory: "Symptoms, defenses, character structure and personality [are regarded] as terms describing the individual's typical interaction which occurs in response to a particular context, rather than as intrapsychic entities" (Jackson 1967, p. 140). By using network analysis techniques, clinical staff have learned to view behavior in terms of a client's location within a network system. The following case illustrates this concept.

> Mr. Davis, a feisty 56-year-old man who was a long-time resident of the Bowery, was the focus of attention at an agency case conference. Initially, there was a tendency to concentrate on Mr. Davis's "addictive" personality and inability to significantly alter his lifestyle. After instituting a network approach, however, it became clear that Mr. Davis was embedded within a social world that perpetuated his drinking and pattern of living. As he noted, "If I stop drinking, I have no friends." His friends and associates were all drinkers but they also provided him with food, money, and assistance in getting to the doctor. He earned extra money by doing odd jobs for flophouse managers or doing errands for other

lodgers. From a network perspective, it was evident that any attempts to alter Mr. Davis's drinking behavior would require the structuring of a new social matrix of nondrinkers to replace the old one.

The advantages of network analysis over the nonempirical approaches to natural groups are most apparent in the organizing of agency programs. A network survey of a target population will enable manpower to be more appropriately assigned on the basis of client-risk categories, geography, and temporality. For example, we found that persons who had smaller networks and fewer network clusters were more at risk for developing psychological symptoms on one-year follow-up (Cohen et al. 1986). These data confirmed our impression that those persons with relatively small, unconnected networks should be targets for more intensive interventions.

With respect to planning the geographic focus of interventions, in our investigation of the single-room occupancy elderly, we found that men had substantially larger networks outside the hotel than did women, whereas women had slightly larger networks within the hotel. Attempts to influence the networks of aged males thus necessitate visiting local taverns (see Dumont 1967), restaurants, betting parlors, and the like. Work with elderly females would entail concentrating efforts within the hotels.

A variety of temporal patterns have been discerned. In studying the unattached elderly living in midtown tenements, we observed that although these individuals had extensive personal networks during the day, they had virtually no contacts during the evening. This withdrawal of the personal support system appeared to be largely responsible for a marked exacerbation of neurotic symptoms in the nighttime (Cohen 1976). An examination of the single-room occupancy aged pointed to a less severe diurnal pattern. Two-thirds of all male and female residents had social contacts in the hotel both during the day and the evening. In contrast, three-fourths of the population had no linkages outside the hotel after dark.

It is therefore necessary to orient programs toward two different subsets of urban elderly—the tenement dwellers and those who reside in single-room occupancy hotels. While those inhabiting tenements require more supportive services in the evening, such programs may be less crucial for a majority of the single-room occupancy hotel elderly.

Network analysis is also useful in establishing relationships between agency personnel and indigenous leaders. Our network research uncovered extensive clustering. Among the elderly hotel residents, more than two-thirds were involved in small groups that ranged from constellations of three persons to "quasi-families" dominated by "mothers" who fed, protected, and set norms for 6 to 11 family members who met in their rooms. Other configurations included those centering around alcohol, gambling, and card playing. Our work with older homeless men indicated that four-fifths of them were engaged in some sort of group formation (Cohen and Sokolovsky 1989). Although many of these groups involved the exchange of alcohol, money, food and emotional support were also characteristically provided.

A number of researchers have developed guidelines for working with natural helpers or leaders (Collins and Pancoast 1976; Froland et al. 1981). Natural helpers are individuals identified by others as being good listeners and helpers who provide social support such as encouragement, reassurance, intimacy, problem-centered services (e.g., housekeeping, errands, cooking), and the alleviation of social isolation (Smith 1975). The advantages of natural helpers are their accessibility, the lack of social stigma in accepting their help, the lack of cost, and the basis for friendship or long-term acquaintanceship (Biegel 1984). Natural helpers can include clergy, nurses, meter readers, pharmacists, physicians, letter carriers, and bus drivers. Those in need turn to these individuals because they are available, are trusted, or are seen as having professional expertise (Biegel 1984). Often they are the first to suspect distress among the frail elderly.

Agency personnel must learn to identify leaders and strong network members so as to furnish them with informal supervision for psychosocial and health problems arising within their networks, information regarding available community resources, and backup services when the informal system cannot cope with a situation. In the consultation model pioneered by Collins and Pancoast (1976), they found that one full-time professional can work with as many as 15 natural helpers.

Use at the client level. In moving to the individual client level, although the techniques mentioned appear in an ordinal fashion, they frequently must be managed simultaneously. 1) The Network Analysis Profile should be completed at the same time as the standard intake data. 2) It should be determined whether the client falls within a vulnerable, high-risk category such as persons with relatively small, unconnected networks. If not, less staff time may be required. 3) An assessment of network strengths and weaknesses must be made. Many networks offer therapeutic protection—medication, food, emotional buttressing—independent of staff support.

Mr. Jones, a rail-thin 66-year-old black male with a history of alcoholism, suffered from impaired mobility and a moderate degree of organic brain syndrome. He lived in a small room in a rundown single-room occupancy hotel in midtown Manhattan. Despite his deficits, he has been able to remain in the community as a result of the assistance he received from three persons: Ms. King, who supplied him with food, clothing, conversation, and emotional sustenance; Mr. Arnold, who occasionally lent him money and food; and Ms. Lee, an elderly sister in the Bronx, who made rare visits to the hotel. An altercation between Mr. Jones and Ms. King abruptly terminated their relationship. Mr. Arnold then took over the responsibility for providing basic necessities to Mr. Jones. A month later, Mr. Arnold unexpectedly left town, thereby effectively extinguishing Mr. Jones's support system. Several days later, a maid found Mr. Jones lying on the floor of his room, severely dehydrated and malnourished. He was hospitalized, and an application was processed for nursing home placement.

A contrasting case was that of Mr. Richardson, a 74-year-old white male with a history of severe emphysema, cardiac disease, and difficulty in ambulating. He lived in the same hotel as Mr. Jones. His life revolved around a stable five-member beer-drinking group and four other individuals who made daily visits to his room for casual conversation. Mr. Richardson was also dependent on Mr. Arnold for groceries and other staples. Nonetheless, when Mr. Arnold left the hotel, Mr. Richardson was still enmeshed in a closely knit social matrix that continued to provide him with emotional support and which undertook the responsibilities of supplying him with his physical necessities.

Merely examining Mr. Jones's and Mr. Richardson's health profiles would have been inadequate for predicting their ability to remain in the community. Clinically, Mr. Richardson's health status was worse than Mr. Jones's. Yet because he was able to receive psychosocial aid through a flexible, interconnected network system, he could remain in a noninstitutionalized environment.

4) When a client presents with a problem, resolution is sought first by utilizing network methods. The clinician must first ascertain whether the client's network is able to alleviate the difficulty. For example, if the individual is nonambulatory, is there someone within his or her network who is available to supply the vital necessities? Or if a person presents with a psychological problem, can his or her network be brought together to provide emotional assistance and solutions to the problem? (See use of the network session developed by Garrison described above.) When no person is available within the client's network to furnish support, contact may be initiated with individuals who have been identified as indigenous helpers.

5) Another approach to solving the client's problem may entail

the involvement of "second-order" linkages. Second-order relationships consist of those persons who are not in direct contact with the client, but who are linked to members of the client's network. Having a large second-order zone is an important resource for potential contacts. Should the "friend of a friend" meet the client, there is a high probability they will become friends (Hammer and Schaffer 1975). Thus second-order contacts may be tapped during periods of stress.

6) The tolerance level of the network must be determined. Some network structures may be able to absorb more stress and to provide more services than others.

> Mr. George Scott is a scraggy, affable 59-year-old chronic schizophrenic. When first seen in his small hotel room, he appeared confused and disheveled, with severe functional deficits in personal hygiene, nutrition, budgeting, and social interaction. Clinical staff support was available only during daytime hours. Network analysis, however, revealed that he was the occasional recipient of services from Ms. Hinds, an older woman with a large personal network which centered around the provision of evening meals. Hence Ms. Hinds, who apparently served a "paraprofessional" function, was enlisted in caring for Mr. Scott during nonstaff hours. In return for a small monthly payment, Ms. Hinds provided Mr. Scott with supper as well as the attendant socialization. In addition, Ms. Hinds encouraged him to take his nighttime medications (his principal dose).

7) It should be ascertained whether any formal services under consideration interfere with extant beneficial services supplied by the informal support system. For example, offering clients loan money may result in the severing of ties with neighbors who lend them money along with considerable conversation and emotional support.

8) An assessment of a client's network should indicate whether any components are in conflict with each other. For instance, one agency may be advocating nursing home placement while a second agency is encouraging community living.

9) For the frail or emotionally unstable client, a rupture in network structure can be especially devastating. It is important to determine whether the client is enmeshed in a network vulnerable to disruption. The viability of high-density clusters is frequently predicated on the presence of one key figure. Should this person become incapacitated or change residence, the network may collapse. Similarly, persons engaged in fragile, low-density, starlike configurations are also vulnerable. In either situation, external (agency) support must be immediately available to assist group members.

Ms. Jean Gans was a small, unkempt, but pleasant 52-year-old white woman with a history of alcoholism and acute schizophrenic reactions. She lived at one of the single-room occupancy hotels serviced by an outreach team. She was identified as a member of the network of Mr. John Roy, a tenant leader, with whom she had a strong relationship. When Mr. Roy announced that he intended to leave the hotel, the outreach staff promptly acted to strengthen their therapeutic contacts with Ms. Gans. She subsequently readjusted her own network, increasing her activities with other members of the broken network as well as with staff members. Similar interventions were made with other vulnerable network members.

10) When indicated, groups oriented toward specific needs or services should be created, e.g., a group for recently widowed women or a group to furnish meals to nonambulatory residents (Collins and Pancoast 1976).

How well do network techniques work? In an experimental service program conducted in one single-room occupancy hotel in which two trained social workers employed the individual-centered network techniques outlined above, we found that they were able to use network intervention with three-fourths of 156 clients who were seen over a 15-month period (Cohen and Adler 1984). Of the 156 clients, slightly more than half were aged 60 and over. Although all problems were supposed to be addressed through a network procedure, only 16% of the interventions for the 519 problems that were presented were successful. An intervention was defined as successful if a specific task was accomplished using a network contact. There were no significant differences in success rates between those under and over the age of 60. Furthermore, no network interventions were employed for approximately one-half of the problems presented. Workers generally did not attempt network interventions if the client had previously resisted or failed at the outset of a network intervention, or in those instances in which the client appeared to be incapable of grasping the network concept. Also, emergency situations sometimes precluded a network intervention.

On the positive side, of those problems treated with a network approach, one-third had successful outcomes and one-third of the sample experienced at least one successful network intervention. Here again, there were no significant differences between age groups. Certain problem areas such as sustenance (e.g., food, loans, medical assistance), new housing, and information and advice had higher success rates, whereas drugs and employment had lower success rates.

Hence, our study indicated that network interventions are not appropriate for every problem or person. Within a particular community, individuals are adept at providing support in some areas but not in others. Not surprisingly, those transactions that were part of a population's cultural world were most likely to yield successful intervention outcomes. For example, the folkways of single-room occupancy hotels involve frequent gossiping and advice-giving, exchange of food or money, and intense concerns about the deterioration of the hotel in a world in which fellow lodgers come and go. Thus, project staff were most successful in those network interventions that involved areas such as offering information and advice, sustenance, finding new housing, and dealing with hotel conditions. On the other hand, many individuals had poor work histories and were less comfortable and adept at helping others with employment problems. Similarly, with respect to drug problems, most hotel residents tended to avoid drug abusers, who generally formed a small subculture within many hotels. Consequently, interest in assisting drug abusers in the course of the project was rather low.

Significantly more network successes were found among the least competent individuals, i.e., those clients who had smaller networks and more physical and mental health symptoms. This may be a consequence of more competent individuals having exhausted their network resources prior to coming to the project staff. They expected and demanded that the project staff provide direct services. If a network intervention was attempted, it may have been done grudgingly within a network that was burnt out. Conversely, clients with fewer personal resources were seemingly less certain that they had adequately utilized their social skills to obtain assistance for a particular problem. They were more disposed to attempt to expand their networks or to try new approaches with their old networks. Hence, their success rates were higher than those of residents who had more personal resources.

Finally, even when the problem area and client profile may be optimal for a network intervention, other factors may intervene to thwart success. Several key factors emerged during the project as obstacles to attempting network interventions in lieu of direct services.

1. Distrust—Many clients were reticent about discussing their personal networks in detail with the project staff. In some cases, they remained guarded because they perceived the workers as being connected with governmental programs.
2. Perceived isolation—Although researchers in the hotel had uncovered an extensive informal network system that provided a

multitude of services, individuals were seemingly unaware of the supportive nature of their social ties. As one staff member observed, "It all added up for the worker to be in a sense searching for something others could not perceive."

3. Confidentiality—For some clients, certain areas (e.g., money) were considered private matters and could only be discussed with an "official" person such as a social worker.
4. Crisis atmosphere—Problems frequently had to be dealt with immediately, and this did not allow adequate time to work with the network.

SUMMARY

We believe that an analysis of the mores of the population, combined with an ongoing assessment of the personal characteristics associated with success, can assist workers to select those problems and clients most amenable to network interventions. Of course, these analyses must be conducted in concert with the further development and refinement of intervention techniques. Moreover, because situational factors, especially problems presenting as crises, emerged as inappropriate for network intervention, successful network interventions must be viewed as an unhurried, long-term effort. The fact that the project staff identified distrust of professionals and a lack of sensitivity to one's personal network as major impediments indicated that considerable rapport and education may be required before a network procedure can be implemented.

The cautionary tone with respect to the use of network interventions reflects the need to avoid touting informal support systems as a quick fix for the provision of services. As the Task Force on Community Support Systems (1978) observed (p. 144), we must guard against using natural supports to justify "public policies which would withhold resources from people to obtain needed professional and formal institutional services." Social network approaches do not eliminate professional staff. Rather, they provide additional roles and contexts in which the clinician can best serve the needs of the older client.

REFERENCES

Antonucci TC: Personal characteristics, social support, and social behavior, in Handbook of Aging and the Social Sciences, 2nd Edition. Edited by

Binstock RH, Shanas E. New York, Van Nostrand Reinhold, 1985, pp 94–128

Barnes JA: Class and committees in Norwegian island parish. Human Relations 7:39–58, 1954

Bengston V: Ethnicity and aging: problems and issues in current social science inquiry, in Ethnicity and Aging. Edited by Gelfand DE, Kutzik AJ. New York, Springer, 1979, pp 9–31

Biegel DE, Shore BK, Gordon E: Building Support Networks for the Elderly. Beverly Hills, CA, Sage, 1984

Boissevain J: Friends of Friends. New York, St. Martin's, 1974

Bott E: Family and Social Networks. London, Tavistock, 1957

Cantor M: Life space and the social support system of the inner city elderly of New York. Gerontologist 15:23–27, 1975

Cohen C: Nocturnal neurosis of the elderly: failure of agencies to cope with the problem. Geriatr Soc 24:86–88, 1976

Cohen C, Adler A: Network interventions—do they work? Gerontologist 24:16–22, 1984

Cohen C, Sokolovsky J: Clinical use of network analysis for psychiatric and aged populations. Community Ment Health J 15:203–213, 1979

Cohen C, Sokolovsky J: Social networks and the elderly: clinical techniques. International Journal of Family Therapy 3:281–294, 1981

Cohen CI, Sokolovsky J: Old Men of the Bowery. New York, Guilford, 1989

Cohen C, Teresi J, Holmes D: Social networks, stress, and physical health: a longitudinal study of an inner-city population. J Gerontol 40:478–486, 1985

Cohen C, Teresi J, Holmes D: Assessment of stress-buffering effects of social networks on psychological symptoms in an inner-city elderly population. Am J Community Psychol 14:75–91, 1986

Collins AH, Pancoast DL: Natural Helping Networks. Washington, DC, National Association of Social Workers, 1976

Dumont MP: Tavern culture, the sustenance of homeless men. Am J Orthopsychiatry 37:938–945, 1967

Froland C, Pancoast DL, Chapman NJ, et al: Helping Networks and Human Services. Beverly Hills, CA, Sage, 1981

Garrison J: Network techniques: case studies in the screening–linking–planning conference method. Fam Process 13:337–353, 1974

Garrison JE, Howe J: Community intervention with the elderly: a social network approach. J Am Geriatr Soc 24:329–333, 1976

Gottlieb BH: Social networks and social support in community mental health, in Social Networks and Social Support. Edited by Gottlieb BH. Beverly Hills, CA, Sage, 1981

Gottlieb BH: Social Support Strategies. Beverly Hills, CA, Sage, 1983

Hammer M, Schaffer A: Interconnectedness and the duration of connections in several small networks. American Ethnologist 2:297–308, 1975

Hammer M, Barrow S, Gutwirth L: A Micro-Social Study of Schizophrenic Ex-Patients in a Community Setting (mimeograph). New York, New York State Psychiatric Institute, 1976

Jackson DD: The individual and the larger contexts. Fam Process 6:139–147, 1967

Mitchell J: Social Networks in Urban Situations. Manchester, England, University of Manchester Press, 1969

Pilisik M, Minkler M: Supportive networks: Life ties for the elderly. Journal of Social Issues 36:95–115, 1980

Smith S: Natural Systems and the Elderly: An Unrecognized Resource. Portland, OR, Regional Research Institute for Human Services, Portland State University, 1975

Snow DL, Gordon JB: Social network analysis and intervention with the elderly. Gerontologist 20:463–467, 1980

Sokolovsky J, Cohen C: Toward a resolution of methodological dilemmas in network mapping. Schizophr Bull 7:109–116, 1981

Task Force on Community Support Systems: Report to President's Commission on Mental Health, Vol 2. Washington, DC, U.S. Government Printing Office, 1978

Thomas PD, Goodwin JM, Goodwin JS: Effect of social support on stress-related changes in cholesterol level, uric acid level, and immune function in an elderly sample. Am J Psychiatry 142:735–737, 1985

Walker KN, MacBride A, Vachon MHS: Social support networks and the crisis of bereavement. Soc Sci Med 2:35–41, 1977

Chapter Six

TIME-LIMITED PSYCHODYNAMIC THERAPY WITH OLDER ADULTS

George Silberschatz, Ph.D., and John T. Curtis, Ph.D.

There has been a long-standing, pervasive bias against psycho-therapy with older adults. Freud (1898, 1905) voiced a common and still prevalent view when he suggested that middle-aged and older adults are not amenable to psychotherapy because they have very limited expectations due to their advanced age, are too set in their ways, and are too rigid characterologically:

> On the one hand, near or above the fifties the elasticity of the mental processes, on which the treatment depends, is as a rule lacking—old people are no longer educable—and, on the other hand, the mass of material to be dealt with would prolong the duration of the treatment indefinitely. (Freud 1905, pp. 258–259)

According to Freud, resistance to treatment among older patients is so great that the therapy would have to go on indefinitely (see also Alexander and French 1946; Fenichel 1945). In the clinical and research literature, the approaches to psychotherapy with older adult patients often reflect tacit acceptance of this bias. This is manifested, for example, in the widespread advocacy and use of medications as the sole or primary ingredient in the treatment of emotional disorders of the elderly (e.g., Busse 1981). This bias is also evident in the prevailing "catastrophic view of aging" (Gutmann 1980; see also, Newton et al. 1984; Steury 1978) and may be seen in some of the emphasis on specialized therapy techniques and modifications in psychother-apeutic practices. For instance, some clinicians have suggested merely providing supportive or palliative measures to older adult psychotherapy patients, implying either that their problems are minor or transitional or that more intensive measures would be wasted effort. (For further discussion, see Blank 1978; Blum and Tross 1980; Butler 1975; Muslin and Epstein 1980; Nemiroff and Colarusso 1985a; Rechtaschaffen 1978; Silberschatz and Curtis, in press).

In contrast to this pessimistic view, other psychodynamic writers have suggested that psychotherapy can be very beneficial to older adults (e.g., Abraham 1919; Colarusso and Nemiroff 1987; Grotjahn 1955; Jung 1933; Kaufman 1937; King 1974; Lazarus 1984; Muslin and Epstein 1980; Myers 1984, 1987; Nemiroff and Colarusso 1985b; Steury and Blank 1978; Zinberg 1964). These authors suggest that elderly patients are no more resistant to change than younger patients. Older patients often are keenly aware of their limited time left to live (Cath 1984; Gould 1972; Neugarten and Datan 1974), and their sense of finitude can be a powerful motivation to overcome resistance and make productive use of psychotherapy. In addition, some investigators have suggested that certain defense mechanisms that might be considered pathological in younger patients serve an adaptive and progressive function in the elderly (Lazarus et al. 1984).

Our studies of time-limited (16 weekly sessions) psychodynamic psychotherapy indicate that older adults with neurotic psychopathology can profit from insight-oriented therapy if the therapist adequately evaluates the patient's treatment goals and devises interventions in accordance with those goals. As a rule, older adults are neither intellectually nor characterologically too rigid to benefit from psychotherapy (see also Berezin 1978; Myers 1984). However, older patients may be more likely to appear fixed, rigid, or defensive in their initial presentation than are younger patients.

We have found that this apparent rigidity and defensiveness often represents what Joseph Weiss (1986) has termed a test of the therapist. According to Weiss, psychopathology stems from pathogenic beliefs or false ideas that are usually unconscious. Pathogenic beliefs are beliefs about oneself and the world that are inferred from experience—typically from traumatic experiences in childhood. These beliefs warn the person who adheres to them about the dangerous consequences of pursuing certain important goals or experiencing certain ideas, wishes, or affects. Patients enter psychotherapy with a plan for solving problems and disconfirming pathogenic beliefs. The patient's plan may be thought of as a strategy, with both conscious and unconscious elements, for disconfirming certain pathogenic beliefs. The strategy may involve both discussion and exploration, as well as testing beliefs in the relationship with the therapist. In testing a pathogenic belief, the patient carries out a trial action intended to provide information about the belief. For example, a patient whose parents were bothered by his autonomous strivings might develop the belief that his autonomy is harmful or upsetting to others, and he thus might stifle certain desires and needs. This patient might test the belief that his autonomous behaviors are harmful by behaving independently in the therapy (e.g., by being late to sessions, coming up with his own insights, ignoring or disagreeing with the therapist's comments) to see if the therapist can comfortably tolerate these behaviors. Conversely, the patient might act excessively reluctant to take initiative in order to test whether the therapist has the same need to control him that he experienced with his parents. Such tests by the patient are part of an active involvement in the therapy (Curtis and Silberschatz 1986; Silberschatz and Curtis 1986).

According to Weiss (1986), when the therapist disconfirms the patient's pathogenic expectations, the test is passed, and the patient is likely to become more productive and involved in the therapeutic work. By contrast, if the therapist confirms the patient's pathogenic belief, the test is failed, and the patient is likely to show signs of discouragement and retreat (see also Curtis and Silberschatz 1986; Silberschatz and Curtis 1986). Our empirical studies of psychotherapy have supported this view; we have found that therapist interventions are most helpful to patients when they are compatible with the patient's plan (Silberschatz et al. 1986) and pass the patient's tests (Bush and Gassner 1986; Silberschatz 1986). A patient is not necessarily consciously aware of the ongoing testing process, and passing tests does not always require the therapist to interpret the genetic origins of the patient's pathogenic beliefs.

The concepts of testing and of the plan compatibility of therapist interventions can broaden our understanding of the process of psychotherapy with older adults and help explain why some older adult patients behave in therapy in a manner that seems to confirm Freud's pessimistic view of their potential for treatment. For instance, we have found that tests in which older patients underestimate themselves or complain about the futility of expecting change at their late stage of life are fairly common. These tests can be difficult to discern (and to pass) when they are expressed subtly. For instance, one patient's frequent request for medications—even though seemingly justified by his complaints of anxiety and insomnia—represented an important test of the therapist. In this particular case, the patient regarded the therapist's acceding to this request as confirmation that he (the patient) should be satisfied with palliative measures rather than exploring and resolving his underlying conflicts. A second patient tested her therapist by describing seemingly appropriate, but very limited, ambitions. This patient experienced the acceptance of these goals by the therapist as confirmation of her unconscious concern that she should allow herself only very limited aspirations. Thus, while the therapist intended to counter any feelings of self-devaluation or discouragement by supporting the patient's stated goals, in so doing, he inadvertently reinforced the patient's pessimism about expecting more.

We now give some clinical examples, drawn from brief dynamic psychotherapies, to illustrate how an apparent resistance can be viewed usefully as a test of the therapist.

A 60-year-old widow, whom we will call "Rita," entered our brief therapy program with the presenting complaint that she was unable to allow herself any pleasure or enjoyment. Rita reported that she had decided recently to take a vacation and had gone so far as to drive to a resort and check in, but then felt she should not stay and had gone home. Rita worked in a middle management position for many more hours than she was paid, frequently going to her job on weekends or even in the middle of the night. When she had time off, she generally felt lost and unable to fill it. At such times, she would usually volunteer to babysit or perform some other chore for one of her adult children.

The therapist learned that Rita had come from a very impoverished background and that her mother had been extremely passive and compliant to her demanding, brutish husband. Rita reported that her mother always looked haggard and had died in her 40s, apparently worn out by the effects of poverty, an abusive husband, and the need to care for more than 10 children (both her own and those of relatives).

In the early hours of therapy, there were frequent, long silences. There were no spontaneous associations, and Rita took no initiative in presenting or discussing issues. When the therapist inquired about her thoughts during the silences, Rita would reply, for example, that she had been thinking about his shoes, and then say no more. Rather than viewing this pattern as a resistance, the therapist regarded Rita's behavior as an important test. That is, Rita identified with her mother's masochism, and she was testing the therapist to see if he needed her to be self-demeaning and lifeless. The therapist interpreted the patient's silence as a reflection of her discomfort over taking control and doing something good for herself. He noted that in the therapy the patient was acting helpless like her mother because she felt uncomfortable about getting more out of life than her mother had. Following this interpretation, the patient began to associate more freely and to explore her conflicts more productively. She also provided confirmation for the therapist's formulation by recalling how her mother, after having a foot amputated, would hop around on one leg, waiting on her healthy but indolent husband.

The preceding example illustrates how an older adult patient may invite the therapist to see him or her as untreatable or to collude with limited expectations for treatment (see also Blum and Tross 1980). We believe that some of the pessimism concerning the treatment of older adults stems from a failure to understand the tests these patients present and, in particular, a tendency to see these patient behaviors as signs of resistance or rigidity rather than as essential parts of the therapeutic process that in fact represent an attempt to work on core issues. However, this begs the question of why an older patient would present these types of tests. As Blum and Tross (1980) noted in their review of the literature on psychotherapy of the elderly, "Several authors have pointed out that the older patient himself often becomes the perpetrator of an ageist mythology" (p. 211).

We see guilt as an important explanatory factor and have found the concept of survivor guilt to be particularly useful in understanding the resistance of older patients to treatment. Niederland (1961) introduced the concept of survivor guilt based on his psychoanalytic and psychotherapeutic work with survivors of the Holocaust. He conceptualized it as a powerful, often unconscious feeling of guilt, together with unconscious fears of punishment, for having survived a calamity in which others suffered or perished. Survivors typically believe that they could or should have helped save a loved one and torment themselves for failing to do so. According to Niederland, survivor guilt does not necessarily originate from unconscious hostile or aggressive impulses; rather, it is based on the survivors' unconscious belief that remaining alive (i.e., surviving) represents a betrayal of those who perished.

The concept of survivor guilt has been further elaborated (Bush 1989; Friedman 1985; Modell 1965, 1971; Weiss 1986) to include experiences of guilt by people who believe that they have better lives than their family members or loved ones. For instance, Modell (1971) noted that survivor guilt is "not confined to particular diagnostic groups, but represents a fundamental human conflict" (p. 340) and thus has universal significance. This elaboration of the survivor guilt syndrome expands upon Freud's model of guilt (Freud 1930), which emphasizes sexual or aggressive wishes in the development of guilt. While survivor guilt may stem from hostile wishes or impulses, it may also originate from a person's love for one's family and from the false conviction that one has inadvertently harmed a love object— for instance, by getting more of the good things in life than a loved one has received. (For a scholarly review and debate of these views see the *Bulletin of the Menninger Clinic*, 53(2) 1989, in which all of the papers focus on this topic.) While survivor guilt is frequently associated with childhood trauma and early modes of cognition (Bush 1989), it should be emphasized that survivor guilt may arise in various ways at any point in the life cycle (see, for example, Friedman 1985; Modell 1971; Niederland 1981).

In our clinical experience we have found older patients to be particularly vulnerable to survivor guilt because they are likely to have witnessed the decline of friends and relatives. A frequently encountered issue in the older patients seen in our brief psychotherapy project is conflict over maintaining or even enhancing one's life after a spouse dies or is disabled (see also Cath 1984; Groves et al. 1984; Settlage et al. 1988).

"Linda" was a 58-year-old secretary who sought treatment following her husband's retirement due to health problems. Throughout their marriage, her husband had taken the lead in structuring their social and family life, and Linda said that she had learned to be dependent upon him. She claimed to have difficulty operating on her own, and she often sought his approval before allowing herself to do things or feel good about what she had done. For instance, she could not enjoy wearing a new dress unless he approved of its purchase. Since his retirement, Linda's husband had been less active in general and particularly at home. Moreover, though he had always been grouchy and demanding, he was more so after stopping work. Linda found him unpleasant and upsetting to be around and worried that some of his pressured and nervous behavior were "rubbing off" on her.

In addition to her relationship with her husband, Linda complained of anxiety and difficulties concentrating. She also worried that she might be forced to retire because of arthritis and was concerned that these problems might make it hard for her to make a good adjustment to retirement. She stated that she wanted to be able to feel enthusiastic and involved without relying on others and "to be able to stand on my own two feet."

It emerged in treatment that Linda had been the favored child in her family. Her only sibling, an older sister, had schizophrenia and had been very troubled as a child. Linda was always more capable and successful than her sister and felt responsible for her. Linda's mother was bright, well-read, and knowledgeable, though she had little schooling. She was an accomplished singer but had never pursued her art, electing instead to devote herself to her husband and his career. She taught Linda to always put one's husband first and behaved that way in her marriage—she always "put him up front and put herself in the background." While her mother was deferring to her husband, Linda felt that she herself was held in too high esteem by her father. He had high expectations of her and often praised her accomplishments. She felt especially uncomfortable when he compared her favorably to her sister.

Linda's problems appeared to represent a form of survivor guilt, stemming from her discomfort as a child about being better off than either her sister or her mother. She had developed the unconscious belief that her successes came at the expense of her mother and her sister and represented a betrayal of them. Thus, she felt that she should not allow herself to have more than or feel better off than her sister or her mother. Her husband's illness provoked a resurgence of these feelings: Linda felt guilty about being better off than he was. Her symptoms of nervousness, anxiety, and poor concentration were clear identifications with her husband, as was her feeling that she might have to retire. In the therapy, her guilt was manifested by her difficulties in clearly conveying her thoughts and insights. In the transference, she worked to disconfirm her pathogenic guilt over enjoying her close relationship with her father; she tested the therapist by initially being very formal and distant from him and gradually feeling warmer and close to him.

A second patient, Millie, was seen in our project following the placement of her husband in a nursing home. He suffered from a degenerative disease which had left him completely helpless. Millie entered therapy to work on this loss and its repercussions (e.g., because of the loss of her husband's income and the expenses involved in his care, she had to seek employment for the first time in her adult life). She was depressed and anxious and very pessimistic about her future. She felt overwhelmed by her problems and the new duties she had assumed and was uncertain how to proceed. One of the central issues she confronted in her therapy was her discomfort over getting on with her life, and not being "paralyzed" like her husband. As was true for Linda, the roots of Millie's survivor guilt were in her early childhood relationships (see below).

Similar guilt feelings over getting on with one's life or prospering can emerge in older adults when their children or grandchildren encounter difficulties.

In the case of Rita, described above, the patient's identification with her masochistic mother was manifested in her relationship with a 30-year-old son who was psychotic. He had married in his teens and was divorced with a 3-year-old child. This son had led a troubled life since adolescence and had been in and out of hospitals most of his adult life. Typically, he shunned psychotherapy and medications and would disappear after a hospitalization, contacting Rita only when in need of money, a place to live, or someone to care for his daughter. Rita suspected that he abused drugs and alcohol. She resented his demands on her and the feeling that he blackmailed her into responding to them by playing on her concerns for his well-being and that of his daughter. She gave him large amounts of money and time in attempts to help him, but he consistently took advantage of her generosity while verbally and physically abusing her for not doing more.

101

Together with her other children, Rita managed to arrange care for her grandchild, but she still felt obligated to respond to her son's ever-increasing demands. Though approaching retirement age, she felt she could not retire because she might not be able to help her son financially without her full salary. The therapist interpreted her excessive feelings of responsibility for her son as a manifestation of Rita's identification with her mother and of her guilt over having a happy life when her son (like her mother) was unhappy. Subsequently, she was able to set appropriate limits on her son's demands.

Another patient, Rose, entered therapy at the suggestion of friends who were concerned that she was giving away all of her money to her grandson. Rose acknowledged to the therapist that her grandson was a ne'er-do-well and that she knew that the money she gave him was being wasted; however, she felt powerless to resist his requests. Her son, the boy's father, had told her to stop giving the grandson money, but to no avail. By the time she entered therapy, this formerly well-to-do widow was in danger of going broke. What emerged in her treatment was that Rose felt guilty about being well off when her grandson was struggling. One way that she worked on her guilt was by actively testing whether the therapist would feel guilty and give in to unreasonable demands. For example, Rose demanded that the therapist extend her hours, call cabs for her, and the like. When he refused her excessive demands, she appeared wounded and acted petulant, but was subsequently able to decline her grandson's requests.

More generally, we have seen a number of older adults who express their survivor guilt by stating that their goals are probably inappropriate or too bold for "an old person."

Because of the financial burden of her husband's illness, Millie (see above) had to find a job. She also wanted to work as a way of maintaining contact with others and as an outlet for her energy and talents. However, she was paralyzed at the thought of seeking employment. Though very bright and articulate, Millie insisted that she was unable to learn new skills or face the rigors of holding a job. Moreover, she stated that society did not want to hire older workers and that she would not be given a chance. When the therapist encouraged her to work, she accused him of being insensitive to her plight (and to the plight of all older women wanting to reenter the work force) and of failing to recognize her limitations.

Millie sought and found employment following interpretations that she felt guilty about being able to work when her husband was not. This dynamic was also linked to Millie's relationship with her mother, a whiny, infantile character who would flee to her parents' house at the slightest difficulty with her husband. As a child, Millie had been accused by her mother of being willful and selfish when she pursued her own interests. In fact, when her parents divorced, mother told Millie that she was leaving father because Millie had been insensitive and too much to deal with. The therapist pointed out that one of the impediments to Millie's seeking employment was her discomfort over being more capable and resilient than her mother and disproving her mother's negative view of her. Thus, Millie's purported helplessness and accusations toward the therapist can be seen as a test of whether the therapist, like her mother, felt she should hold herself back. It may also have served as a test to see how the therapist would handle the sorts of accusations Millie herself had experienced.

The feelings of older people about their aspirations and goals can also be influenced by what they witnessed occurring with their parents in old age (Cath 1984). For instance, they may question whether they can or should handle old age and death better than their parents.

A 59-year-old man was referred for psychotherapy by his physician because of various physical complaints that appeared to be psychosomatic. The patient initially spoke in detail about his physical symptoms and then noted that on several occasions he inexplicably had broken into tears. He had no immediate ideas about these incidents and did not connect them with his physical complaints. However, at the end of the first session, when it was explained to him that his physical symptoms might be manifestations of emotional concerns, he wondered aloud whether his crying jags might be related to concerns about hating his father. At the beginning of the second session, he reported that he had been thinking a great deal about his past. Among a number of memories, he recalled that as a child he was always very frightened of his father, who was often physically violent. He felt that this fact would in some way prove very important in understanding his physical problems. He also spontaneously wondered whether his symptoms were in some way serving as a punishment. In the third session, he said that while talking with his wife he had realized that he might fear going insane because both his father and sister had had serious psychiatric problems. His father had begun acting patently "strange" a number of years before his death at age 70. Upon further reflection, the patient associated the beginning of his symptoms with having reached the same age his father was when he began showing signs of psychosis. With further exploration, it became apparent that a significant issue for this patient was his guilt about entering his later years without suffering emotionally like his father and sister had.

While we believe that guilt is a significant factor influencing the feelings and behavior of older adults, we certainly do not mean to suggest that other factors do not play important and often limiting roles in the treatment of the elderly (see also Myers 1984, 1987; Steury and Blank 1978). The loss of physical and cognitive functioning that often accompanies aging can place realistic limits on what will be accomplished in therapy. Also, as a group, older adults are more likely to have suffered significant, often irreplaceable losses (Zetzel 1965). Ignoring these realistic limits and experiences can do the older adult as much disservice as underestimating potential. However, it is important to examine the impact of these realistic events in a case-specific manner to determine their true impact on and meaning for the patient. For instance, research has shown that the meaning of loss—and thus its impact—for the older adult is often much different (less traumatic) than for a younger adult (see, for example, Neugarten and Datan 1974).

Our experience with and studies of older adults in psychotherapy has led us to conclude that as a group they are as amenable to treatment as younger adults. Indeed certain concomitants of aging seem to assist the older patient in treatment. A lifetime of experiences—including the resolution of other problems—can provide older adults with a better perspective on and greater optimism about current problems. As illustrated in the case examples, the problems of older adults often are related to trauma that occurred earlier in life. The distance from these original trauma can make them easier to explore and understand. Similarly, having fulfilled different roles can provide the older patient with an understanding of other's feelings and behaviors that is often not available to younger adults.

> For example, an older adult patient was traumatized in her early relationship with her mother. Her mother acted severely wounded whenever the patient displayed any independence or defiance, and the patient grew up feeling that she could easily devastate others unless she was very careful. She generalized these feelings to other people and relationships in her life and was plagued with excessive worries about how she might or might not have injured someone by something she had said or done. Because of her fears of hurting others she was generally mousy and undemonstrative, even in situations where she was clearly being mistreated. Once this patient became aware of the basis of her concerns, she was able to employ her experiences as a mother to disconfirm her beliefs about her ability, as a child, to harm her mother. Having been in both roles of the relationship (mother and daughter) enabled her to recognize and correct distortions that had developed when she did not have this perspective.

Different perspectives that develop with aging can also help the older adult patient in psychotherapy. For instance, the sense of limited remaining time (Cath 1984; Gould 1972; Neugarten and Datan 1974) can speed up the therapeutic work; the older patient has less time to waste and will often confront and work through issues in a more bold and aggressive manner than a younger patient. In part this may reflect the different issues confronted by older and younger adults, for example, the nature of separation and autonomy issues that are common among younger adults may require extended periods of time to work through. Nevertheless, it is our impression that the older adult—as a consequence of experience, different perspectives, and a sense of time—generally works in therapy as well as, if not better than, a younger adult and is capable of achieving as good a result as his or her younger counterpart.

Because of the biases that have long existed in the psychological and psychiatric literature concerning the elderly, therapists may underestimate (albeit in subtle or insidious ways) these patients and thereby fail significant initial tests. When therapists fail these tests, patients may drop out of treatment, and therapists may conclude that older patients are too resistant and cannot benefit from psychotherapy. However, when these important tests are passed, as in the above case examples, we have observed striking changes in patients, such as their becoming less depressed and revealing more daring and ambitious goals. Our studies suggest that it is not necessary to educate elderly patients about therapy or to systematically modify the treatment procedures. Rather, we have found that what is most predictive of successful therapy is the ability of the therapist to ascertain and respond appropriately to the patient's goals for therapy and to help the patient disconfirm pathogenic beliefs.

REFERENCES

Abraham K: The applicability of psycho-analytic treatment to patients at an advanced age (1919), in Selected Papers on Psychoanalysis. New York, Basic Books, 1953, pp 312–317

Alexander F, French TM: Psychoanalytic Therapy: Principles and Application. New York, Ronald Press, 1946

Berezin MA: Psychodynamic considerations of aging and the aged: an overview, in Readings in Psychotherapy With Older People (DHEW Publ No ADM-78-409). Edited by Steury SR, Blank ML. Washington, DC, U.S. Government Printing Office, 1978, pp 21–29

Blank ML: Raising the age barrier to psychotherapy, in Readings in Psychotherapy With Older People (DHEW Publ No ADM-78-409). Edited by Steury SR, Blank ML. Washington, DC, U.S. Government Printing Office, 1978, pp 62–67

Blum JE, Tross S: Psychodynamic treatment of the elderly: a review of issues in theory and practice, in Annual Review of Gerontology and Geriatrics, Vol 1. Edited by Eisdorfer C. New York, Springer, 1980, pp 204–234

Bush M: The role of unconscious guilt in masochism. Bull Menninger Clin 53:97–107, 1989

Bush M, Gassner S: The immediate effect of the analyst's termination interventions on the patient's resistance to termination, in The Psychoanalytic Process: Theory, Clinical Observation, and Empirical Research. Edited by Weiss J, Sampson H, Mount Zion Psychotherapy Research Group. New York, Guilford, 1986, pp 299–320

Busse EW: Therapy of mental illness in late life, in American Handbook of Psychiatry, Vol 7, 2nd Edition. Edited by Arieti S, Brodie HKH. New York, Basic Books, 1981, pp 505–526

Butler RN: Psychiatry and psychology of the middle-aged, in Comprehensive Textbook of Psychiatry, 2nd Edition. Edited by Freedman AM, Kaplan HI, Saddock BJ. Baltimore, Williams & Wilkins, 1975, pp 2390–2404

Cath SH: A psychoanalytic hour: a late-life awakening, in Clinical Approaches to Psychotherapy With the Elderly. Edited by Lazarus LW. Washington, DC, American Psychiatric Press, 1984, pp 1–14

Colarusso CA, Nemiroff RA: Clinical implications of adult developmental theory. Am J Psychiatry 144:1263–1270, 1987

Curtis JT, Silberschatz G: Clinical implications of research on brief dynamic psychotherapy, I: formulating the patient's problems and goals. Psychoanalytic Psychology 3:13–25, 1986

Fenichel O: The Psychoanalytic Theory of Neurosis. New York, Norton, 1945

Freud S: Sexuality in the aetiology of the neuroses (1898), in The Standard Edition of the Complete Psychological Works of Sigmund Freud, Vol 3. Translated and edited by Strachey J. London, Hogarth Press, 1959, pp 261–285

Freud S: On Psychotherapy (1905), in The Standard Edition of the Complete Psychological Works of Sigmund Freud, Vol 7. Translated and edited by Strachey J. London, Hogarth Press, 1959, pp 257–268

Freud S: Civilization and its discontents (1930), in The Standard Edition of the Complete Psychological Works of Sigmund Freud, Vol 21. Translated and edited by Strachey J. London, Hogarth Press, 1961, pp 57–145

Friedman M: Toward a reconceptualization of guilt. Contemporary Psychoanalysis 21:501–547, 1985

Gould RL: The phases of adult life: a study in developmental psychology. Am J Psychiatry 129:521–531, 1972

Grotjahn M: Analytic psychotherapy with the elderly. Psychoanal Q 42:419–427, 1955

Groves L, Lazarus LW, Newton N, et al: Brief psychotherapy with spouses of patients with Alzheimer's disease: relief of the psychological burden, in Clinical Approaches to Psychotherapy With the Elderly. Edited by Lazarus LW. Washington, DC, American Psychiatric Press, 1984, pp 37–53

Gutmann DL: Psychoanalysis and aging, in The Course of Life: Psychoanalytic Contributions Toward Understanding Personality Development, Vol III: Adulthood and the Aging Process (DHHS Publ No ADM-81-1000). Edited by Greenspan SI, Pollock GH. Washington, DC, U.S. Government Printing Office, 1980, pp 489–517

Jung CG: Modern Man in Search of a Soul. New York, Harcourt, Brace & World, 1933

Kaufman MR: Psychoanalysis in late-life depressions. Psychoanal Q 6:308–335, 1937

King P: Notes on the psychoanalysis of older patients. Journal of Analytical Psychology 19:22–37, 1974

Lazarus LW (ed): Clinical Approaches to Psychotherapy With the Elderly. Washington, DC, American Psychiatric Press, 1984

Lazarus LW, Groves L, Newton N, et al: Brief psychotherapy with the elderly: a review and preliminary study of process and outcome, in Clinical Approaches to Psychotherapy With the Elderly. Edited by Lazarus LW. Washington, DC, American Psychiatric Press, 1984, pp 15–35

Modell AH: On having the right to a life: an aspect of the super-ego's development. Int J Psychoanal 46:323–331, 1965

Modell AH: The origin of certain forms of pre-oedipal guilt and the implications for a psychoanalytic theory of affects. Int J Psychoanal 52:337–346, 1971

Muslin H, Espstein LJ: Preliminary remarks on the rationale for psychotherapy of the aged. Compr Psychiatry 21:1–12, 1980

Myers WA: Dynamic Therapy of the Older Patient. New York, Jason Aronson, 1984

Myers WA: Dreams of mourning and separation in older individuals, in The Interpretation of Dreams in Clinical Work. Edited by Rothstein A. Madison, CT, International Universities Press, 1987, pp 105–123

Nemiroff RA, Colarusso CA: The literature on psychotherapy and psychoanalysis in the second half of life, in The Race Against Time: Psychotherapy and Psychoanalysis in the Second Half of Life. Edited by Nemiroff RA, Colarusso CA. New York, Plenum, 1985a, pp 25–43

Nemiroff RA, Colarusso CA (eds): The Race Against Time: Psychotherapy and Psychoanalysis in the Second Half of Life. New York, Plenum, 1985b

Neugarten BL, Datan N: The middle years, in American Handbook of Psychiatry, Vol 3. Edited by Arieti S. New York, Basic Books, 1974, pp 592–608

Newton NA, Lazarus LW, Weinberg J: Aging: biopsychosocial perspectives, in Normality and the Life Cycle. Edited by Offer D, Sabshin M. New York, Basic Books, 1984, pp 230–285

Niederland WG: The problem of the survivor. Journal of the Hillside Hospital 10:233–247, 1961

Niederland WG: The survivor syndrome: further observations and dimensions. J Am Psychoanal Assoc 29:413–426, 1981

Rechtschaffen A: Psychotherapy with geriatric patients: a review of the literature, in Readings in Psychotherapy With Older People. (DHEW Publ No ADM-78-409). Edited by Steury SR, Blank ML. Washington, DC, U.S. Government Printing Office, 1978, pp 45–61

Settlage CF, Curtis JT, Lozoff M, et al: Conceptualizing adult development. J Am Psychoanal 36:347–369, 1988

Silberschatz G: Testing pathogenic beliefs, in The Psychoanalytic Process: Theory, Clinical Observation, and Empirical Research. Edited by Weiss J, Sampson H, Mount Zion Psychotherapy Research Group. New York, Guilford, 1986, pp 256–266

Silberschatz G, Curtis JT: Clinical implications of research on brief dynamic psychotherapy, II: how the therapist helps or hinders therapeutic progress. Psychoanalytic Psychology 3:27–37, 1986

Silberschatz, G, Curtis JT: Research on the psychodynamic process in the treatment of older persons, in Psychodynamic Research Perspectives on Development, Psychopathology, and Treatment in Later Life. Edited by Miller NE. New York, International Universities Press (in press)

Silberschatz G, Fretter PB, Curtis JT: How do interpretations influence the process of psychotherapy? J Consult Clin Psychol 54:646–652, 1986

Steury SR: The later years: a psychological perspective, in Readings in Psychotherapy With Older People. (DHEW Publ No ADM-78-409). Edited by Steury SR, Blank ML. Washington, DC, U.S. Government Printing Office, 1978, pp 3–7

Steury SR, Blank ML (eds): Readings in Psychotherapy With Older People (DHEW Publ No ADM-78-409). Washington, DC, U.S. Government Printing Office, 1978

Weiss J: Part I: theory and clinical observations, in The Psychoanalytic Process: Theory, Clinical Observation, and Empirical Research. Edited by Weiss J, Sampson H, Mount Zion Psychotherapy Research Group. New York, Guilford, 1986, pp 3–138

Zetzel ER: The dynamics of the metapsychology of the aging process, in Geriatric Psychiatry. Edited by Berezin MA, Cath SH. New York, International Universities Press, 1965, pp 109–119

Zinberg NE: Psychoanalytic considerations of aging. J Am Psychoanal Assoc 12:151–159, 1964

PSYCHOPHARMACOLOGICAL AND PSYCHOTHERAPEUTIC TREATMENTS IN DIFFERENT SETTINGS

Chapter Seven

DIAGNOSIS AND PHARMACOLOGICAL TREATMENT OF DEPRESSION IN OLDER PATIENTS

Steven P. Roose, M.D.

O lder patients are most often referred for psychopharmacological consultations because of two disorders, depression and Alzheimer's disease. A discussion of the diagnosis and treatment of Alzheimer's disease is outside the scope of this chapter. Rather, I will focus on affective disorder in the patient over 65, the particular considerations for making this diagnosis in the older patient, and the pharmacokinetic factors that significantly affect pharmacological treatment in this group.

PREVALENCE

Though few epidemiological studies have specifically focused on the incidence or prevalence of affective disorder in the patient population over the age of 65, the available data are consistent with the belief that depression is one of the most frequently occurring serious illnesses in the elderly population. A prevalence rate of affective disorder from 2% to 10% has been reported, and one European study estimated the lifetime risk (up to age 80) of severe depressive illness as 17% for women and 8% for men (Butler 1975a, 1975b; Essen-Moller et al. 1956; Gurland 1976). It must be remembered, however, that if a study is reporting depressive symptoms only and not differentiating between symptoms and the syndrome of depression, then there is a tendency to overestimate significantly the prevalence of psychopathology because transient and mild depressive phenomena will be overrepresented (Georgotas 1983). Another statistic that can be used to

111

help estimate the rate of serious affective disorder in the elderly population is the incidence of suicide. Certainly not all people who commit suicide have affective disorder, but multiple studies have shown a high correlation between suicide and affective disorder (Guze and Rubins 1970; Pokorny 1964; Rubins et al. 1959; Weissman 1974). Though in the period 1975–1977 people 65 and older comprised approximately 11% of the population, this same group disproportionately accounted for 25% of the suicides (Busse and Pfeiffer 1977; Sendbuehler 1977).

DIAGNOSIS

The diagnostic criteria for a major depressive episode according to DSM-III-R mandate that a patient must have either a depressed mood or a pervasive loss of interest or pleasure (American Psychiatric Association 1987). In addition, this must be accompanied by at least four of the following symptoms: significant weight loss or decreased appetite, insomnia or hypersomnia, psychomotor agitation or retardation, marked fatigue or loss of energy, feelings of worthlessness or excessive or inappropriate guilt, a diminished ability to think or concentrate, recurrent thoughts of death, or suicide attempts. Although DSM-III-R recognizes that modification of the diagnostic criteria for a major depressive episode is necessary when assessing a pediatric population, there has been no formal consideration of whether the diagnostic criteria for depression should be modified when evaluating an older population. Yet it is a long-standing clinical belief that the older depressed patient may not experience a depressed mood, but rather have a multitude of somatic complaints such as abdominal pain, generalized muscle weakness and pain, headaches, and arthralgia. The predominance of somatic symptoms often observed in elderly depressed patients gave rise to the concept of "masked" depression; that is, the "true" depressed mood of the elderly patient is converted into somatic symptoms and the consequent barrage of somatic complaints serves to mask the underlying depression. This concept implies that the somatic complaints of the patient are not "real." However, after the development of the idea of masked depression, there was more appreciation for the fact that depressive syndrome is a systemic illness with significant effects on multiple organ systems, including the cardiovascular, gastrointestinal, neuroendocrine, and musculoskeletal. Therefore, rather than considering somatic complaints as the patient's inarticulate substitutions for depressed mood, they should be considered symptoms of the depressive syndrome itself; they are not masking anything but are to be taken at face value.

Another phenomenological consideration that has specific importance to the older population is the presence of delusions as part of a depressive syndrome. Approximately 25% of patients hospitalized for treatment of melancholic depression have delusional depressions (Glassman and Roose 1981). This diagnosis has significant implications because it is known that delusional depressions do not respond to standard antidepressants alone and require either a combination of antidepressants and antipsychotics or electroconvulsive therapy (ECT) (Roose and Glassman 1988). Effective treatment is especially critical since patients with delusional depressions have an increased risk of suicide compared to nondelusional patients (Roose et al. 1983). A number of studies have reported that as patient age increases, so does the incidence of delusions as part of a depressive syndrome (Hordern et al. 1963; Meyers et al. 1984; Post 1982; Spicer et al. 1973).

A third important consideration in the diagnosis of affective disorder in older people is concurrent serious medical illness. This problem has two components: 1) the differential diagnosis of affective disorder in the older patient, namely whether the affective disorder is a manifestation of an occult illness with a known etiology, e.g., hypothyroidism or pancreatic cancer, and 2) whether the patient has a chronic medical condition that has caused the affective disorder. With respect to the first situation, all older patients with a diagnosis of affective disorder should have a thorough physical examination and certain laboratory tests, including electrocardiogram, blood chemistries and electrolytes, blood count, and thyroid studies. With respect to the second consideration, studies report a 10% to 50% rate of affective disorder in patients with various chronic medical conditions such as emphysema, angina, and arthritis (Moffie and Paykel 1975). Though treatment response of depression in this setting has not been systematically studied, there is general consensus that if a significant affective disorder is present, there should be a trial of standard antidepressant treatment. This is especially true for patients with cardiovascular disease since there are data to indicate that among these patients, those who are depressed have a higher rate of morbidity and mortality from their cardiovascular illness than those who are not depressed (Roose et al. 1989). This observation is compatible with the long-standing observation that patients with depression have a higher than expected rate of death from sudden cardiovascular events (Malzberg 1937). Thus, there is a complicated and bidirectional relationship between depression and underlying medical conditions, particularly cardiovascular problems, and this set of complicated circumstances is frequently present in the older patient.

Furthermore, the presence of a chronic medical illness often means

113

the patient is taking one or more medications, e.g., antihypertensives and/or oral hypoglycemics. A number of medications have been reported to affect mood adversely. Thus, the patient's current medication regimen should be scrupulously reviewed during the initial diagnostic evaluation. In addition, if an antidepressant is prescribed for a patient who is already taking one or more medications, the clinician must be aware of possible drug-drug interactions.

Because many prominent symptoms of depression in the older patient are somatic, e.g., sleep disturbance, fatigue, focal pain, it is not surprising that patients will often first consult their medical doctor. In the recent past it was not uncommon that patients with such complaints were examined, told there was nothing physically wrong, and sent out of the office with a prescription for a benzodiazepine. However, with increasing awareness of the prevalence of and criteria for diagnosis of major affective disorder, an accurate diagnosis of depression is now often made by the primary care physician. Currently, a more pervasive problem with the older patient is a misconception about the relationship between aging and depression; namely, the belief that it is "understandable" that an older patient is depressed considering the external realities of his or her life, which generally include failing health, restricted mobility, and the loss of friends and relatives. Rather than "empathic," this misconception often results in the clinician not initiating treatment for this serious illness.

PHARMACOLOGICAL TREATMENT OF DEPRESSION

Multiple studies over the past two decades have definitively documented the effectiveness of various types of medication in the treatment of depression. The most extensive and conclusive data bear on the use of the tricyclic antidepressants. Like all psychotropic medications except for lithium, the tricyclics are lipid-soluble drugs. Two key pharmacokinetic factors determine the fate of an oral dose of a lipid-soluble drug: volume of distribution and metabolism. The volume of distribution for a lipid-soluble drug is significantly related to body mass. In clinical terms that means, for example, that prescribing 150 mg of imipramine for a 100-pound woman is very different from ordering 150 mg of imipramine for an obese 300-pound man. With respect to metabolism, it must be remembered that the critical process in the metabolism of a lipid-soluble drug is the conversion of the lipid-soluble metabolite that can then be excreted from the body. In the metabolism of a tricyclic, this conversion is accomplished by hydroxylation of the carbon in the "two" position of the ring, a step that is catalyzed by a cytochrome P450 reductase enzyme in the liver (Glassman and Perel 1973). Enzyme capacity is a genetically determined trait and thus identical twins will have the same amount of enzyme and first-degree relatives more similar amounts of enzyme compared to nonrelatives, but the interindividual variation in enzyme capacity is considerable (Glassman and Perel 1973).

Given these differences in volume of distribution and metabolism, it is not surprising that fixed oral doses of tricyclic antidepressants produce widely varying plasma levels when given to randomly selected patients. This observation, among others, led to the hypothesis that there is an important relationship between tricyclic plasma level and clinical outcome. Studies in the United States and Scandinavia have established the relationship between tricyclic plasma level and clinical outcome for three of the most widely used drugs: imipramine, nortriptyline, and desmethylimipramine (Asberg et al. 1971; Glassman et al. 1977; Nelson et al. 1982). Thus, the current standard of optimal tricyclic treatment is to administer a therapeutic plasma level of drug for an adequate period of time.

When considering the treatment of the older depressed patient, there are two questions about tricyclic treatment: 1) Is the plasma level necessary for response in the older patient lower compared with younger patients? 2) Does the aging process significantly affect either of the pharmacokinetic factors that influence attaining a therapeutic level of tricyclic? With respect to the first question, indirect data from a number of studies and, more recently, direct data from studies by Nelson and colleagues (1985) have documented that depressed patients over the age of 65 require the same level for therapeutic response as younger patients.

However, compared with younger patients, older patients usually require a lower oral dose to reach a therapeutic plasma level as a consequence of the influence of aging on a number of pharmacokinetic factors. With respect to volume of distribution, it is known that elderly patients tend to be smaller than younger patients (Greenblatt et al. 1982). Furthermore, as humans age, although total body weight may not increase significantly, lean body mass is reduced and percent of body fat rises (Bruce et al. 1980; Novak 1972). This change in total body fat significantly increases the volume of distribution for lipid-soluble drugs, which in turn prolongs drug half-life (Greenblatt et al. 1980, 1981). In addition, most psychotropic drugs bind to a plasma protein, in particular serum albumin. For example, with a tricyclic antidepressant, 95% of the plasma level is bound to albumin and only 5% of the concentration is free drug; but it is the free drug component

115

that is critical in terms of drug activity (Glassman and Perel 1973). A number of studies have reported that in elderly persons serum albumin levels decrease by 15% to 25%, and the less albumin available for drug binding, the greater the free drug component (Bender et al. 1975; Hayes et al. 1975; Schumacher 1980). This may translate into increased adverse effects, especially in a vulnerable population.

It is known that aging affects the metabolism and excretion of most medications. With respect to hepatic metabolism, hepatic blood flow decreases significantly with age, which theoretically should mean decreased hepatic metabolism (Bender 1965; Geokas and Haverback 1969). However, the interindividual differences in enzyme capacity are still the most important determinants of hepatic metabolism even in the elderly, and so, in the absence of hepatic disease, it is hard to draw any conclusions about the clinical impact of aging on the hepatic component of drug metabolism.

The impact of aging on renal excretion is well studied and has significant implications. All parameters of renal function, including glomerular filtration rate and creatinine clearance, decreased significantly with age (Papper 1978; Rowe and Besdine 1982). This fact has implications for drugs whose clearance is partly or entirely a function of renal excretion. For example, it has been shown that with increasing age the oral dose of lithium required to maintain a constant therapeutic level may decrease by as much as one-half (Hewick and Newbury 1976).

In summary, a number of pharmacokinetic parameters must be considered when treating the older depressed patient. However, none of these factors precludes the use of antidepressant medication. Rather, if proper adjustments are made, the elderly depressed patient can, for the most part, be safely and effectively treated.

ADEQUATE TREATMENT

Despite the many effective treatments available, depression is still often inadequately treated. A number of studies have demonstrated that, even in university medical centers, as many as 50% of patients with major affective disorder receive an inadequate dose or inadequate duration of a pharmacological agent (Keller et al. 1986). This has led to an inflated rate of nonresponders or treatment-resistant depressions (Schatzberg et al. 1986).

This problem of inadequate treatment is even more prevalent in the older depressed patient and is not simply due to failure to make an accurate diagnosis of depression or to recognize that older patients need therapeutic levels of drugs. The problem of increased sensitivity of the elderly to the medication, as manifested by a higher rate and severity of side effects, can significantly contribute to less-than-optimal medication treatment. For example, a major concern in the elderly population is the cardiovascular effects of these drugs (Roose and Glassman 1989). In depressed patients with preexisting cardiac disease, a number of considerations govern the use of antidepressant medication. However, even in the medically healthy older depressed patient, orthostatic hypotension (systolic blood pressure falls when going from a lying to a standing position) is a frequent and serious complication (Glassman et al. 1979). Though the orthostatic effect of tricyclic antidepressants is a phenomenon that occurs in both younger and older depressed patients, clearly the consequences are greater in the elderly depressed patient (Roose et al. 1981) who is more likely to become symptomatic and fall. The consequences of a fall in an elderly depressed patient can be quite serious, as evidenced by a study reporting that a patient over the age of 65 taking antidepressants has a significantly higher risk of hip fracture than a patient of comparable age not taking this class of drugs (Ray et al. 1987).

Another special problem in the elderly depressed patient is that he or she may have an increased sensitivity to the anticholinergic effects of the tricyclic antidepressants. The nuisance side effects induced by the anticholinergic effect of these drugs are dry mouth and constipation. However, it is the more serious anticholinergic effect, namely confusion, that is particularly prominent in the elderly depressed patient. A depressed patient who may have some underlying but not yet manifest Alzheimer's disease may become significantly confused when exposed to the anticholinergic effect of tricyclics.

Thus, older patients treated with tricyclics may be more sensitive to side effects and pharmacokinetic factors may lower the oral dose needed to reach a therapeutic plasma level. But depression is a prevalent illness and has a significant morbidity and mortality when left untreated. Though pharmacological treatment is potentially more complicated in the older patient, the medications are no less effective in an elderly depressed population and the illness should be aggressively treated. All these considerations taken together have led to the solid clinical advice that when treating older depressed patients with medication "start low, go slow, but go all the way."

PARTIALLY TREATED DEPRESSION

Though the tricyclic antidepressant medications, when used at proper levels, are generally effective for the treatment of depression in all age groups, there nonetheless remains a group of patients who are at best only partially improved. Their pattern of improvement will often reflect the nonspecific pharmacological effects of the tricyclics and thus the patient may report improved sleep, decreased agitation or anxiety, and somewhat increased appetite. However, a core of depressive symptoms, albeit somewhat attenuated, will clearly persist. For example, the patient's mood will still be somewhat depressed, he or she will experience a minimum of pleasure and, in short, clearly will not return to the premorbid self. Though the patient has not recovered, the urgency for relief that is experienced by both the physician and patient is reduced. The consequent danger is that the partially treated depression will be accepted as the patient's new "baseline." It is only after waiting an appropriate period of time for the medication to take full effect and recognizing that, despite robust improvement in the first couple of weeks, it may take further time for the patient to work through the impact of having had such a major illness, that a diagnosis of partially treated depression can be made.

There is a generic countertransference problem that increases the risk of not recognizing a partially treated depression in the older patient. That is the misconception that some chronic depressive symptoms are a "natural reaction to the aging process." As with the initial diagnosis of depression in the elderly, the therapist's fantasies and, often, ignorance of what it is to become old can be a significant obstacle to the patient obtaining proper treatment.

A partial response or no response at all to the first trial of antidepressants naturally raises the question of what constitutes a reasonable sequence of somatic treatment of depression that balances the pursuit of cure versus the risk of side effects. If a patient has not responded to a therapeutic plasma level of a tricyclic, the next step is to augment the tricyclic by adding one of three medications: lithium, thyroid, or stimulants. Of the three, only lithium has demonstrated effectiveness when compared to placebo in double-blind studies. Initial studies by de Montigny et al. (1983) and subsequent larger studies by Henninger et al. (1983) have shown that when lithium is added to tricyclics in the plasma level range of 0.4 to 1.0 mEq/l, 50% of the patients will have a robust response within 3 weeks.

If lithium augmentation of tricyclics is not effective, there are three other treatments with some data to suggest effectiveness. There are no data, however, to suggest in what sequence these treatments should be administered; that decision would depend on individual circumstances. There are data showing that, with classical melancholia, monoamine oxidase (MAO) inhibitors can produce a therapeutic effect in patients who have failed to respond to tricyclics. Of particular note is that the largest study on this topic was done in patients over the age of 70, thus further demonstrating that not only can MAO inhibitors be effective in this population, but they are also safe and well tolerated (Georgotas et al. 1983a).

The data on the new specific serotonergic drugs are more limited. At this point there are only anecdotal case reports or very small studies that have attempted to demonstrate a therapeutic effect of the serotonergic drugs in patients who have failed to improve on tricyclics (Lingjaerde et al. 1983; Nolen et al. 1988; Nystrom and Hallstrom 1987; Potter et al. 1981). More extensive information on this group of drugs bears not on their effectiveness, but rather on their side effect profile compared to the other standard antidepressant medications. Specific serotonergic drugs, for example fluoxetine, do not have the significant anticholinergic effect of the tricyclics or MAO inhibitors and this can have special importance for older patients who are vulnerable to anticholinergic-induced confusional states. Furthermore, the reported lack of orthostatic blood pressure effect could avoid the most severe cardiovascular problem associated with the tricyclics (Fisch 1985). However, two considerations must be taken into account when comparing the side effect profile of the serotonergic drug to the standard tricyclic. First, to date the side effects of the serotonergic drugs have not been systematically studied in an older patient population, but rather have been determined in a younger depressed population free of medical disease. Whether the serotonergic drugs will be as well tolerated in older patients who have multiple medical problems and/or whether there will be significant drug interactions common to the older population remains to be seen. Second, it is not that the serotonergic drugs are without side effects, but rather that their side effect profile is different from the standard tricyclics. For example, serotonergic drugs induce significant nausea, sleep disruption, and anxiety, but not dry mouth or urinary obstruction (Wernicke 1985).

Finally, it must be remembered that electroconvulsive therapy, the oldest treatment known for affective disorder, still remains one of the safest and most effective. In recent studies by Prudic and co-workers it has been demonstrated that electroconvulsive therapy is effective in 40% to 50% of depressed patients who have failed adequate trials of antidepressant medications (Prudic and Sackeim 1990). Thus, even in a medication-resistant depressed population, ECT is a treatment with potential benefit and should not be avoided in the older patient because of undue fear of side effects or complications.

In summary, as with the younger patient, the older depressed patient should not be labeled treatment-resistant or treatment-refractory, nor should the patient or the physician be satisfied with a partial response until all safe and effective treatments have been judiciously administered. On the other hand, if standard treatments have not been effective, one must caution against the practice of "emptying the medicine chest" and exposing the patient to one treatment after another—treatments that may have little evidence to support their efficacy, but carry a risk of significant side effects.

CONCLUSION

The diagnosis and psychopharmacological treatment of affective disorder in the older patient require attention to phenomenological and pharmacokinetic considerations unique to this age group. Furthermore, treating the elderly can bring forth countertransference problems that can significantly impede the therapeutic process. Nonetheless, if sufficient attention is given to these issues, older depressed patients can, for the most part, be safely and effectively treated with antidepressant medications.

REFERENCES

American Psychiatric Association: Diagnostic and Statistical Manual of Mental Disorders, 3rd Edition, Revised. Washington, DC, American Psychiatric Association, 1987

Asberg M, Cronholm B, Sjoqvist F, et al: Relationship between plasma level and therapeutic effect of nortriptyline. Br Med J 3:331–334, 1971

Bender AD: The effect of increasing age on the distribution of peripheral blood flow in man. J Am Geriatr Soc 13:192–198, 1965

Bender AD, Post A, Meier JP, et al: Plasma protein binding of drugs as a function of age in adult human subjects. J Pharm Sci 64:1711–1713, 1975

Bruce A, Andersson M, Arvidsson B, et al: Body composition: prediction of normal body potassium, body water, and body fat in adults on the basis of body height, body weight, and age. Scand J Clin Lab Invest 40:461–473, 1980

Busse EW, Pfeiffer E: Behavior and Adaptation in Late Life, 2nd Edition. Boston, Little, Brown, 1977

Butler RN: Psychiatry and the elderly: an overview. Am J Psychiatry 132:893, 1975a

Butler RN: Psychotherapy in old age, in American Handbook of Psychiatry, Vol 5, 2nd Edition. Edited by Arieti S. New York, Basic Books, 1975b

de Montigny C, Cournoyer G, Morrissette R, et al: Lithium carbonate addition in tricyclic antidepressant-resistant unipolar depression. Arch Gen Psychiatry 40:1327–1334, 1983

Essen-Moller E, Larsson H, Uddenberg EC, et al: Individual traits and morbidity in a Swedish rural population. Acta Psychiatr Scand Suppl 100:1–160, 1956

Fisch C: Effect of fluoxetine on the electrocardiogram. J Clin Psychiatry 46:42–44, 1985

Geokas MC, Haverback BJ: The aging gastrointestinal tract. Am J Surg 117:881–892, 1969

Georgotas A: Affective disorders in the elderly: diagnostic and research considerations. Age Ageing 12:1–10, 1983

Georgotas A, Friedman E, McCarthy M, et al: Resistant geriatric depressions and therapeutic response to monoamine oxidase inhibitors. Biol Psychiatry 18:195–205, 1983

Glassman AH, Perel JM: The clinical pharmacology of imipramine. Arch Gen Psychiatry 28:649–653, 1973

Glassman AH, Roose SP: Delusional depression: a distinct clinical entity? Arch Gen Psychiatry 38:424–427, 1981

Glassman AH, Perel JM, Shostak M, et al: Clinical implications of imipramine plasma levels for depressive illness. Arch Gen Psychiatry 34:197–204, 1977

Glassman AH, Bigger JT Jr, Giardina EGV, et al: Clinical characteristics of imipramine-induced orthostatic hypotension. Lancet 1:468–472, 1979

Greenblatt DJ, Allen MD, Harmatz JS, et al: Diazepam disposition determinants. Clin Pharmacol Ther 27:301–312, 1980

Greenblatt DJ, Divoll M, Puri SK, et al: Clobazam kinetics in the elderly. Br J Clin Pharmacol 12:631–636, 1981

Greenblatt DJ, Sellers EM, Shader RI: Drug disposition in old age. N Engl J Med 306:1081–1088, 1982

Gurland BJ: The comparative frequency of depression in various adult age groups. J Gerontol 31:283–292, 1976

Guze SB, Robins E: Suicide and primary affective disorders. Br J Psychiatry 117:437–438, 1970

Hayes MJ, Langman MJS, Short AH: Changes in drug metabolism with increasing age: phenytoin clearance and protein binding. Br J Clin Pharmacol 2:73–79, 1975

Heninger GR, Charney DS, Sternberg DE: Lithium carbonate augmentation of antidepressant treatment; an effective prescription for treatment-refractory depression. Arch Gen Psychiatry 40:1335–1342, 1983

Hewick DS, Newbury PA: Age: its influence on lithium dosage and plasma levels. Br J Clin Pharmacol 3:354, 1976

Hordern A, Holt NG, Burt CG, et al: Amitriptyline in depressive states: phenomenology and prognostic considerations. Br J Psychiatry 109:815–825, 1963

Keller MB, Lavori PW, Klerman GL, et al: Low levels and lack of predictors of somatotherapy and psychotherapy received by depressed patients. Arch Gen Psychiatry 43:458–466, 1986

Lingjaerde O, Bratfos O, Bratlid T, et al: A double-blind comparison of zimelidine and desipramine in endogenous depression. Acta Psychiatr Scand 68:22–30, 1983

Malzberg B: Mortality among patients with involution melancholia. Am J Psychiatry 93:1231–1238, 1937

Meyers BS, Kalayam B, Mei-Tal V: Late-onset delusional depression: a distinct clinical entity? J Clin Psychiatry 45:347–349, 1984

Moffie HS, Paykel ES: Depression in medical inpatients. Br J Psychiatry 126:346–353, 1975

Nelson JC, Jatlow PI, Quinlan DM, et al: Desipramine plasma concentration and antidepressant response. Arch Gen Psychiatry 39:1419–1422, 1982

Nelson JC, Jatlow PI, Mazure C: Desipramine plasma levels and response in elderly melancholic patients. J Clin Psychopharmacol 5:217–220, 1985

Nolen WA, van de Putte JJ, Dijken WA, et al: Treatment strategy in depression, I: nontricyclic and selective reuptake inhibitors in resistant depression: a double-blind partial crossover study on the effects of oxaprotiline and fluvoxamine. Acta Psychiatr Scand 78:668–675, 1988

Novak LP: Aging, total body potassium, fat-free mass, and cell mass in males and females between ages 18 and 85 years. J Gerontol 27:438–443, 1972

Nystrom C, Hallstrom T: Comparison between a serotonin and a noradrenaline reuptake blocker in the treatment of depressed outpatients: a crossover study. Acta Psychiatr Scand 75:377–382, 1987

Papper S: Clinical Nephrology. Boston, Little, Brown, 1978

Pokorny AD: Suicide rates in various psychiatric disorders. J Nerv Ment Dis 139:499–506, 1964

Post F: Affective disorders in old age, in Handbook of Affective Disorders. Edited by Paykel E. New York, Guilford, 1982

Potter WZ, Calil HM, Extein I, et al: Specific norepinephrine and serotonin uptake inhibitors in man: a crossover study with pharmacokinetic, biochemical, neuroendocrine, and behavioral parameters. Acta Psychiatr Scand Suppl 290:152–170, 1981

Prudic J, Sackeim HA: Refractory depression and electroconvulsive therapy, in Treatment Strategies for Refractory Depression. Edited by Roose SP, Glassman AH. Washington DC, American Psychiatric Press, 1990, pp 109–128

Ray WA, Griffin MR, Schaffner W, et al: Psychotropic drug use and the risk of hip fracture. N Engl J Med 316:363–369, 1987

Robins E, Murphy DE, Wilkinson RH Jr, et al: Some clinical considerations in the prevention of suicide based on a study of 134 successful suicides. Am J Public Health 49:888–899, 1959

Roose SP, Glassman AH: Delusional depression, in Depression and Mania. Edited by Georgotas A, Cancro R. New York, Elsevier, 1988, pp 76–85

Roose SP, Glassman AH: Cardiovascular Effects of Tricyclic Antidepressants in Depressed Patients. Journal of Clinical Psychiatry Monograph Series No 7. 1989

Roose SP, Glassman AH, Siris SG, et al: Comparison of imipramine- and nortriptyline-induced orthostatic hypotension: a meaningful difference. J Clin Psychopharmacol 1:316–319, 1981

Roose SP, Glassman AH, Walsh BT, et al: Depression, delusions, and suicide. Am J Psychiatry 140:1159–1162, 1983

Roose SP, Glassman AH, Dalack GW: Depression, heart disease, and tricyclic antidepressants. J Clin Psychiatry 50(7) (suppl):12–17, 1989

Rowe JW, Besdine EW: Health and Disease in Old Age. Boston, Little, Brown, 1982

Schatzberg AF, Cole JO, Elliott GR: Recent views on treatment-resistant depression, in Psychosocial Aspects of Nonresponse to Antidepressant Drugs. Edited by Halbreich U, Feinberg SS. Washington DC, American Psychiatric Press, 1986, pp 94–109

Schumacher GE: Using pharmacokinetics in drug therapy, VII: pharmacokinetic factors influencing drug therapy in the aged. Am J Hosp Pharm 37:559–562, 1980

Sendbuehler J, Goldstein S: Attempted suicide among the aged. J Am Geriatr Soc 25:245–248, 1977

Spicer CC, Hare EG, Slater E: Neurotic and psychotic forms of depressive illness: evidence from age incidence in a national sample. Br J Psychiatry 123:535–541, 1973

Weissman MM: The epidemiology of suicide attempts, 1960 to 1971. Arch Gen Psychiatry 30:737–746, 1974

Wernicke JF: The side effect profile and safety of fluoxetine. J Clin Psychiatry 46:59–67, 1985

Chapter Eight

THERAPEUTIC INTERVENTIONS BY GERIATRICIANS

Jeffrey N. Nichols, M.D., Cheryl A. Walters, M.D., and Morton D. Bogdonoff, M.D.

The evaluation and treatment of primary psychiatric disorders and the psychiatric complications of primary medical disorders play a large part in the practice of the average nonpsychiatric geriatrician. Physicians from every specialty may from time to time be called to assist in the care of psychiatric patients. Primary care physicians all know the large percentage of ambulatory care visits that are primarily for the treatment of neurotic conditions and personality disorders (Hankin et al. 1982). But the trained geriatrician is particularly likely to be consulted for those cases in which frail elderly individuals face medical and social problems with immediate or potential neuropsychiatric complications. With the recent elevation of geriatrics to certificate status by the American Board of Internal Medicine and the American Board of Family Practice, and with the gradual increase in divisions of geriatrics within hospitals and medical schools, the role of the geriatrician in the care of such patients is likely to increase. There are now over 2,500 certified geriatricians in the United States and several thousand others who practice primarily in geriatrics but are technically ineligible for certification, choose not to be tested, or have failed to pass.

SOME COMMON VARIETIES OF PATIENT DISORDERS SEEN BY GERIATRICIANS

Cognitive Disorders

The geriatrician is frequently asked to evaluate patients with disorders of cognition. The elderly patient with gradual onset of confusion or memory loss might be brought to the geriatrician for diagnosis in the setting of a private office or hospital outpatient clinic, or even at the time of nursing home admission. The acute onset of confusion and abnormal behavior in an elderly patient may lead to geriatric consultation. Alternatively, the geriatric clinician may observe changes in mental status in a patient who has been followed in the past for other medical problems. The differential diagnosis of delirium from dementia or pseudodementia is at the heart of the practice of most geriatricians. Indeed, recent Medicare regulations for the preadmission screening of nursing home residents for mental illness or mental retardation would allow this to be done by a psychiatrist, neurologist, or certified geriatrician.

Depression

A second major involvement of geriatricians in the psychiatric care of elderly patients is the evaluation and treatment of depression. Changes in appetite, libido level, weight, sleep, concentration, or energy level are frequently brought first to the attention of the geriatrician. Initial evaluation by the geriatrician is particularly common when multiple medications and diagnoses are present or when the patient or family has already established a therapeutic relationship with the physician. One study found an 11.5% prevalence of major depression and a 23% prevalence of other depressive syndromes in elderly patients hospitalized for medical illness (Koenig et al. 1988). There was a higher risk for those individuals with more severe medical problems. The prevalence of depression in nursing homes rises to 35% (Lewis et al. 1985). The geriatrician frequently treats the fatal illness of one marital partner and the depression of the survivor.

Chronic Psychiatric Disorders

A smaller, but still significant portion of a typical geriatric practice involves the medical care of patients with chronic psychiatric disorders that are continuing into senescence. The prevalence of alcoholism in elderly patients has grown with an aging population. More than one-third of the members of Alcoholics Anonymous are over the age of 50 (Gorbien 1989). Alcohol abuse enters into the differential diagnoses of many classic geriatric syndromes including frequent falls, confusional states, osteoporosis, and "failure to thrive." Manic-depressive illness, schizophrenia, personality disorders, and anxiety disorders are also seen in older people. The geriatrician frequently provides continuing care for these problems among multiple, inter-related medical problems.

Somatic Complaints

Finally, physicians in every aspect of practice encounter patients with somatiform disorders. Although these patients are no more common among the elderly population (indeed, physicians since Hippocrates have noted that elderly patients complain less than younger ones), they represent a particularly troublesome group for geriatricians (Hippocrates, *Aphorisms*). This is because the frequency of multiple and chronic illnesses and of atypical presentations of physical ailments in this age group makes the exclusion of organic etiologies for these patients' symptoms especially difficult (Hodkinson 1973; Wilson et al. 1962).

MEANS OF PATIENT REFERRAL

Many elderly patients self-refer to the geriatrician. Consultations from other medical specialties are also common, although there is still some reluctance for general internists and family practitioners to accept geriatrics as a legitimate subspecialty. Similarly, Medicare will usually not accept billing from a geriatrician for a patient already being followed by an internist or a general practitioner. Referrals for behavioral problems in elderly patients frequently come from concerned family members or worried caregivers. Many institutions (adult homes, health-related or skilled nursing facilities) maintain relationships with geriatricians as providers of primary care or as consultants. Social agencies such as home care agencies, senior centers, or religious groups may request an evaluation of a frail elderly person who appears to be failing. Within the maze of involved people and agencies, it is sometimes difficult to separate treating the patient from treating the complainant.

EVALUATION

The primary task for the geriatrician is usually the exclusion of organic illnesses that present with or exacerbate preexisting psychiatric symptoms. DSM-III-R (American Psychiatric Association 1987) criteria for the diagnosis of both dementia and major depression require the exclusion of other organic etiologies. Over 80% of patients over the age of 65 have one chronic ailment while 50% have two or more (Shamoian 1983). An extraordinarily long list of medical problems may present primarily with central nervous system manifestations in elderly patients (see Table 8-1). Although more careful studies have dimmed the initial enthusiasm for the search for "reversible dementia" (Barry and Moskowitz 1988; Clarfield 1988), there is still some yield from assessment. Indeed, every older person presenting with the recent onset of psychiatric symptoms deserves a careful medical workup.

The key to medical evaluation by the geriatrician is a comprehensive history and physical examination, followed by a directed laboratory evaluation. Of these elements, the history is by far the most important. It should include a chronology of the current problem; a delineation of past medical and social landmarks; diet; and a comprehensive review of symptoms, prior response to treatment, and past and present medications. The examiner must not be embarrassed to ask about alcohol use, drug use, or sexual practices.

Patients over the age of 65 consume 25% of all medications prescribed by physicians and one and one-half times as many over-the-counter medications as prescription drugs (Lamy 1980). An extraordinarily large number of medications in common use have a potential for side effects, as is clear from Table 8-2. In fact, drug intoxication is believed to be the most common cause of delirium in elderly patients (Lipowsky 1989). Many medications, including antibiotics, diuretics, and antineoplastics, have been associated with mental status changes in isolated case reports.

There are over 600 medications with antimuscarinic side effects available in the United States. Many of these are nonprescription drugs used for the treatment of conditions as varied as asthma, muscle spasms, and diarrhea (Peters 1989). Their atropinelike, anticholinergic, or parasympatholytic side effects include dry mouth, urinary retention, memory loss, confusion, hallucinations, agitation, and paranoia. The potential for additive effects from polypharmacy should be obvious. Because of age-related and degenerative changes in the central cholinergic system, elderly patients are especially sensitive to such toxic effects.

Many geriatricians request a "brown bag" evaluation in an initial screening. This consists of asking the patient to empty her or his medicine cabinet into a container and bring the contents into the office. Many patients need more than one bag, and suitcases are not unusual. Each medication is reviewed in turn, and the patient is asked to describe how frequently it is used and for what specific indications (if known). Elderly persons often cannot read the small type on pill containers and rely on their memories as a guide to dosage and frequency. Patients may be taking both the trade and generic forms of the same medication, which have been prescribed by different practitioners, and/or continuing medications that the physician intended to stop. Multiple studies have shown that while elderly patients have no greater degree of noncompliance than younger ones, their increased sensitivity to medication and their higher percentage of medication usage make them more vulnerable to the effects of noncompliance (Stewart and Caranasos 1989). A home visit is also an ideal opportunity for medication review, particularly for patients who may be reluctant to show the physician medications obtained from other sources. The home visit may also reveal unexpected hints of behavioral disorganization or alcohol abuse.

Case Illustration

A social service agency requested evaluation of a client because of recent weight loss and complaints of malaise. This 84-year-old German Jewish refugee had a 40-year history of recurrent depression since her sister's suicide. She had recently developed significant visual loss due to macular degeneration. In the initial interview conducted in the living room of her apartment, the patient denied all medication use except an occasional sleeping pill. The interview revealed confusion, disorientation to time, a depressed affect, and loss of recent and remote memory. When the examiner moved to the bedroom to conduct the physical examination, he found at the bedside multiple half-filled pill containers containing diphenhydramine, Sominex, Sleep Eze, temazepam, and secobarbital with amobarbital. The diphenhydramine came from a local practitioner and the temazepam prescription from the patient's ophthalmologist, whereas the secobarbital with amobarbital had been prescribed 4 years previously by a physician who had subsequently retired. The patient was uncertain which of these medications she had taken. All medications were removed, and the patient's mental status cleared. Her appetite improved, and she returned to her baseline mild depression.

The medical history of the cognitively impaired adult is usually provided by a member of the family. Many clinicians are cautious about accepting family assessments of mental status, particularly with respect to the onset and course of dementing illnesses. Hospital house staff complain that families often inaccurately describe elderly relatives as being mentally intact prior to the onset of an acute illness that has produced confusion and memory loss. This can, in turn, lead to unnecessary and invasive neurological evaluations. Denial may, of course, play a role here, as does the fear that a loved one will be ignored or considered senile. Often, however, the apparent misinformation comes from a failure to take an effective history coupled with

Table 8-1. Medical conditions presenting with psychiatric symptoms

Category	Examples
Nutritional deficiencies	Thiamine (Wernicke-Korsakoff), niacin (pellagra), vitamin B_{12}, folic acid, pyridoxine
Primary intracranial processes	Tumors (primary or metastatic), normal pressure hydrocephalus, cerebrovascular accident, multi-infarct dementia, posttraumatic syndromes, seizures, subdural hematoma, degenerative dementias (Alzheimer's, Parkinson's, Pick's, or Wilson's disease; progressive supranuclear palsy, Shy-Drager syndrome)
Endocrine	Hyperthyroidism, hypothyroidism, hyperparathyroidism, hypoparathyroidism, diabetes mellitus, diabetes insipidus, pheochromocytoma, Cushing's syndrome, Addison's disease, estrogen replacement, hypertestosteronism
Metabolic	Metabolic acidosis, metabolic alkalosis, dehydration, hypernatremia, hyponatremia, hypokalemia, hypoxemia, hypercalcemia, hypocalcemia, hyperphosphatemia, hypomagnesemia, porphyria
Infection	Delirium (regardless of cause, with or without fever), bacterial or fungal meningitis, encephalitis, human immunodeficiency virus dementia, neurosyphilis, brain abscess, cerebral malaria, Lyme disease, rheumatic arteritis, subacute bacterial endocarditis, Whipple's disease, babesiosis, typhus, Jacob-Kreutzfeld disease

Toxic	Ethanol and drug intoxications or withdrawal, carbon monoxide, heavy metals
Cardiovascular	Hypertensive encephalopathy, congestive heart failure, myocardial infarction, arrhythmias, aortic stenosis, murantic endocarditis, cardiopulmonary bypass
Hematologic	Iron deficiency anemia, hypoplastic anemias, hyperviscosity syndrome (multiple myeloma, macroglobulinemia, or leukemic crisis), paraneoplastic syndromes, tumor lysis syndrome, polycythemias, disseminated intravascular coagulation
Rheumatologic	Polyarteritides (nodosa, temporal, or giant cell; granulomatous), vasculitis (rheumatoid arthritis, systemic lupus erythematosis), sarcoidosis, cryoglobulinemia, immune complex disease
Miscellaneous	Fecal impaction, urinary retention, pain (regardless of etiology), sensory deprivation (intensive care unit psychosis), amyloidosis, acute pancreatitis, dialysis, portal-systemic shunt, fat emboli, postoperative states

Table 8-2. Common nonpsychiatric medications with psychiatric side effects

Drug	Usual indication	Reaction
Acyclovir	Herpetic infection	Hallucinations, confusion
Albuterol	Bronchodilator	Paranoia, hallucinations
Amantadine	Parkinsonism, influenza	Hallucinations, delusions, nightmares, mania, exacerbation of schizophrenia
Amphetamines	Narcolepsy, drug of abuse	Bizarre behavior, anxiety, agitation, paranoia
Anticonvulsants	Seizure disorder	Toxic encephalopathy, depression, delirium, agitation
Antihistamines	Allergic reactions	Delirium, anxiety (particularly in combination)
Atropine and anticholinergics	Parkinsonism, preanaesthesia, antispasmodics, peptic ulcer, nasal congestion, asthma (may be included in eye drops, skin patches, or inhaled preparations)	Confusion, memory loss, hallucinations, paranoia, agitation
Baclofen	Muscular spasm	Hallucinations, paranoia (usually with medication withdrawal)
Beta-blockers (propranolol, atenolol, timolol, etc.)	Hypertension, essential tremor, angina, glaucoma, arrhythmia (may be included in eye drops)	Depression, confusion, paranoia
Bromocriptine	Parkinsonism	Mania, delusions (may persist several weeks after drug discontinued)

Captopril	Hypertension, heart failure	Anxiety, hallucinations, mania
Clonidine	Hypertension	Depression, delirium
Codeine	Pain, cough	Dysphoria and depression, euphoria, nightmares, anxiety, paranoia
Corticosteroids	Numerous, including chronic obstructive pulmonary disease, rheumatic diseases, dermatologic conditions, cancer chemotherapy	Mania, depression, confusion, paranoia, catatonia
Diazepam	Muscle relaxant	Rage, hostility, depression, amnesia, paranoia
Digitalis	Heart failure, arrhythmia	Nightmares, euphoria, confusion, amnesia, aggression, depression (especially at high serum levels)
Disopyramide	Cardiac arrhythmia	Agitation, panic, depression
Ephedrine	Ear, nose, and throat symptoms	Hallucinations, paranoia
Halothane	Anesthesia	Depression (postoperative period)
H2 receptor antagonists (cimetidine, famotidine, ranitidine)	Acid peptic diseases	Hallucinations, delirium, depression, mania, bizarre behavior
Ketamine	Anesthesia	Nightmares, hallucinations, delusions
Levodopa	Parkinsonism	Delirium, depression, agitation, hypomania, paranoia, nightmares
Methyldopa	Hypertension	Depression, amnesia, psychosis

continued

Table 8-2. Common nonpsychiatric medications with psychiatric side effects—*continued*

Drug	Usual indication	Reaction
Metoclopramide	Hiatal hernia, diabetes, gastroparesis	Mania, depression
Narcotics	Pain	Nightmares, anxiety, euphoria, depression, paranoia, hallucinations
Nifedipine	Angina, hypertension	Irritability, agitation
Nonsteroidal anti-inflammatories (ibuprofen, indomethacin, naproxen, sulindac)	Arthritis, analgesia	Paranoia, depression, anxiety, hostility, confusion
Prazosin	Hypertension, heart failure	Depression, hallucinations
Procaine derivatives	Anesthesia (may be combined with other medications)	Panic, confusion, psychosis, agitation (particularly with procaine penicillin G)
Quinidine	Cardiac arrhythmia	Confusion, agitation
Reserpine	Hypertension	Depression
Salicylates	Analgesia	Agitation, confusion (at high serum levels)
Theophylline	Bronchodilator	Anxiety, mania, withdrawal, mutism (at high serum levels)

Source. Adapted from Abramowitz 1989.

ignorance on the part of the family as to the course of normal and pathological aging. Physicians should be aware that significant memory loss is often accepted as the norm by families of octo- and nonagenarians. Many geriatricians prefer a functional approach to obtaining mental status histories from families. Shopping, cooking, managing a checkbook, reading, visiting with friends, or calling friends on the telephone are all tasks that require considerable mental alertness. Questions about the patients' capacity to perform these tasks will provide information about chronic dementia and significant sensory losses. By contrast, a lifelong history of functional impairment or eccentric behavior should provoke a search for underlying diagnoses.

The physical examination may elicit new information or enable one to test out hypotheses developed from the history. The physical examination should include a detailed neurological examination to detect focal deficits and other signs of organic disease, including frontal release signs, coarse tremor, ataxia, asterixis, and myoclonus. Evaluations of hearing and vision are also an essential part of the neurological examination. Formal mental status testing can give important clues to differentiate functional from organic disorders. Careful attention should be paid to orthostatic changes in pulse and blood pressure and to the status of the cardiovascular system. Routine laboratory work should be done, including complete blood count, sedimentation rate, SMA 20, thyroid function tests, VDRL, vitamin B_{12} level, urinalysis, chest X ray, and stool testing for occult blood. Other tests such as an electrocardiogram, computed tomography scan or magnetic resonance imaging of the head, electroencephalogram, barium enema, lumbar puncture, angiography, or brain biopsy, or tests for drug levels or arterial blood gases may be indicated, based on the results of the history and physical examination or as a screening procedure prior to the initiation of medication.

The process of medical evaluation is important not only to exclude diagnoses of organic illness, but also to evaluate comorbid conditions that may significantly affect the psychiatric diagnosis and treatment. The patient with severe hearing loss is not likely to be a good candidate for psychotherapy, regardless of the psychiatric diagnosis. Particular somatic symptoms, such as constipation, palpitations, or anorexia, may be related to the presence of another illness and thus may not be appropriate parameters by which to follow the response to treatment of a concomitant psychiatric disorder. The use of particular psychiatric medications may have to be avoided because of a patient's inability to tolerate cardiac, genitourinary, or neurological side effects.

With elderly persons, it is frequently important to keep the patient's overall prognosis in mind when determining the course of treatment. The individual with end-stage chronic lung disease or the bedridden cardiac patient lacks the life expectancy to undertake a prolonged course of therapy of any type. Wheelchair-bound patients may be unable to come to the office regularly for treatment or monitoring. The approach taken with the cancer patient who has 3 months to live will necessarily be different from that taken with the one who has a high likelihood of attaining 5-year survival.

THERAPEUTICS

Medication Evaluation

The geriatrician's initial approach to therapy is a natural consequence of the evaluation process. Possible or probable underlying medical etiologies, where they exist, must be approached directly. Many of these can be corrected quickly. Potentially confounding or problematic medications should be withdrawn. This may often involve the substitution of other medication with less potential for neuropsychiatric side effects (as, for example, in switching from a beta-blocker to quinidine to control cardiac arrhythmia). This process is not without some degree of risk for patients with complex or severe medical problems. Unfortunately, most elderly depressed hypertensive patients have primary depressions rather than medication reactions.

Case Illustration

A 74-year-old retired schoolteacher with known Alzheimer's disease was brought to the office by her husband because of 3 days of agitation and pacing. The patient's other chronic medical problem was urinary incontinence from bladder spasms, which were well controlled with oxybutynin. Five days previously the patient had developed upper respiratory symptoms, which her husband treated with Actifed and vitamin C. On physical exam she was febrile to 101°F, tachycardic at 96 beats per minute, and quite agitated and restless, plucking at her clothing. Her lungs were clear. The Actifed was withdrawn. Her fever was controlled with acetaminophen. Over the next 2 days, her agitation gradually resolved.

The Interaction Between Medical and Psychiatric Problems

The interrelation between medical and psychiatric problems is often quite complex. Feelings of hopelessness may lead the patient to reject taking medication. If the medication in question happens to be thyroid hormone replacement, for one example, the resulting metabolic derangement will exacerbate the depression. The mildly depressed patient with arthritis may have his or her feelings of depression intensified by the pain of an arthritic flare-up, particularly when physicians and family treat this attack as "just a part of growing old." Such treatment seems to validate the patient's own emotional linkage between the inevitability of aging and what is perceived as necessary pain and loss. The presence of a major depression may also lead to a failure to consult a physician or to actual physical immobility, with the consequent development of contractures and a further loss of function. A short course of a nonsteroidal anti-inflammatory drug might be an initial treatment for the depression.

Reversing Treatable Problems

The key function of the geriatrician is to reverse that which is reversible. Maximizing the patient's independence and function may involve the appropriate referral to other specialties or to allied professions, such as physical therapy, audiology, or optometry. Correction of visual and auditory deficits may often play an important adjunctive role in the treatment of depression; additionally, it may help to reduce paranoid ideation in paraphrenia and to improve cognition and behavior in the delirious or demented patient.

Accurate medical information may also help to relieve anxiety. Elderly people generally share our society's false notions of the aging process. The presence of benign memory loss, an attack of bursitis, or a new diagnosis of a chronic condition such as diabetes or hypertension may be perceived as the beginning of a process of inevitable mental and physical decline. Specific information about diagnosis and prognosis, along with refutation of the myths of aging, may be useful in treating or preventing reactive depression.

Case Illustration

An 88-year-old woman was admitted to a nursing home because of inability to care for herself at home due to severe osteoarthritis. She was tearful during the admission exam, which proceeded slowly due to her profound hearing loss as well as her monosyllabic answers to questions. She described a 40-pound weight gain over the last year, which she blamed on inactivity and an excellent appetite. She took no medications because friends had assured her "there's no cure for arthritis." She also described poor sleep, including episodes of waking at night, which she blamed on arthritis. On admission to the home, she was placed on aspirin, started on a physical therapy program, and fitted for a hearing

137

aid. Within 2 months she was walking freely with a walker and was a talkative participant at social events in the home. After 3 months she called her doctor to request a weight reduction diet.

Environmental Therapy

Beyond the medical model, psychiatric problems in geriatric care are frequently susceptible to environmental therapy. Social isolation may be addressed through referral to existing community supports. These may include activity programs, senior citizens centers, Golden Age or retiree clubs, volunteer activities or senior volunteer corps, Alcoholics Anonymous, or appropriate intergenerational activities for the mobile elderly. The homebound or nearly homebound elderly may benefit from visiting neighbor or telephone contact programs; the Visiting Nurse program; scheduled home visits by the physician; or homebound programs from the parish, church, or synagogue. Where appropriate, a program of physical or occupational therapy at home can enhance physical functioning while decreasing social isolation. Electronic alarm devices worn on the body, which can be used to call for assistance in case of emergency, are available in many communities through hospitals or commercial services. These may decrease nocturnal anxiety. Homemaker services for the physically limited may lead to a cleaner and more pleasant home environment, more nutritious meals, and a greater frequency of social interaction.

Case Illustration
The daughter of an 84-year-old widow requested reevaluation of her mother, who was becoming withdrawn, losing weight, and calling long distance several times a day or in the middle of the night to complain of being sick without any specific symptoms. Ten years previously, the patient had suffered a small stroke with residual moderate memory loss. She had, however, been extremely healthy since, taking no medications and visiting her physician only for an annual physical examination. The patient's account of her illness was confused and repetitious; she emphasized her belief that she was going to die and asked for help. Her apartment was noted to be disorganized. Piles of newspapers and unopened mail cluttered all available surfaces. The refrigerator contained moldy food. Physical examination of the patient revealed a recent 15-pound weight loss and impaired vision. She appeared in otherwise good health, and screening laboratory values were still normal. The patient was referred to an ophthalmologist, who diagnosed glaucoma with severe loss of visual acuity. Pilocarpine drops controlled intraocular pressure but did not improve her vision. Both the daughter and the patient refused psychiatric evaluation or antidepressant medication. The daughter hired a homemaker for 6 hours a day, 7 days a week. The homemaker

prepared and served lunch and dinner, which she shared with the patient. The apartment was cleaned. The homemaker and patient took a daily walk to shop together. The daughter arranged to visit weekly to assist her mother with mail, bills, and other tasks of personal and financial management. The patient regained her lost weight, and her physical complaints disappeared.

Environmental therapy may involve referral to another level of care. The adult home, health-related facility, or nursing home may provide a structured environment, activities, and social contacts. These are crucial for demented elderly persons who live alone and are poor candidates for home services.

Primary Psychiatric Care by the Geriatrician

Geriatricians are frequently providers of conventional primary psychiatric services to elderly patients. Much of the care that family physicians have traditionally given to younger patients, notably short-term family therapy and family conferences, may be useful with the elderly. This is applicable particularly when the older patient's behavior is more distressing to the family than to the patient. Marital counseling for the elderly couple may be done individually or jointly. Psychotherapy addressed to coping with chronic or terminal illness is appropriately combined with the medical visit for that illness. Indeed, the medical visit is frequently an excuse for the real purpose of the appointment. This useful fiction satisfies the physician who may not think of himself or herself as a psychotherapist, the patient who accepts "doctor" visits as a regular occurrence, and the third-party payer who readily reimburses "medical" services.

Assistance with the grieving process is commonly provided through a series of visits designed to address outstanding health issues of the survivors. Such issues are frequently neglected during the stress of the terminal illness of a spouse or loved one. Attention to future needs has the positive effect of turning one's attention away from the past while time is available to deal with unresolved issues involving the deceased. This may be particularly important when the survivor has had a close relationship with the physician during a prolonged or terminal illness and would suffer the double loss of the loved one and the physician.

Finally, the geriatrician is frequently forced into the role of gero-psychiatrist when appropriate psychiatric services are unavailable. Psychiatric services on a less-than-emergency basis are generally unavailable to the homebound elderly. Many small nursing homes have little or no available psychiatric services, especially in parts of the country where shortages of psychiatrists exist. Alcohol, drug abuse, and sex therapy clinics are rarely designed to accommodate the special needs of older clients. Medicare has payment limits for psychiatric services, which are much more restrictive than those for medical services.

In addition, referrals to psychiatric services are often rejected by the patient or the family. Notions of the stigma of mental illness are extremely common among elderly people, especially in the generation born before World War I. While rejecting any emotional etiology for their symptoms, patients may accept medications like trazodone or doxepin to stimulate appetite or promote sleep. Patients or families who are willing to accept the terms nervous, depressed, or confused from a family physician may still see psychiatrists as treating people who are "crazy." These psychiatry-resistant attitudes can persist even in the face of extremely bizarre or paranoid behavior. Explanations for inappropriate behavior that suggest chemical imbalances in the brain may be more readily acceptable than the suggestion of psychiatric intervention, with its still resilient stereotype of the bearded Freudian analyst with his couch, employing psychosexual dynamic models on the elderly patient. Facing these resistances, most geriatricians proceed to treat directly, using standard medications in adjusted doses.

The essence of geriatrics is multidisciplinary care. As America's population ages, and as the medical profession increasingly recognizes the prevalence of depression and other treatable psychiatric illnesses within the aging population, the possibilities for closer collaboration between geriatricians and geropsychiatrists will grow. The dichotomy of mind and body may be at times a useful construct for the younger patient, but it is a dangerous fallacy for the older one.

REFERENCES

Abramowitz M (ed): Drugs that cause psychiatric problems. Med Lett Drugs Ther 31:113–118, 1989

American Psychiatric Association: Diagnostic and Statistical Manual of Mental Disorders, 3rd Edition, Revised. Washington, DC, American Psychiatric Association, 1987

Barry PP, Moskowitz MA: The diagnosis of reversible dementia in the elderly. Arch Intern Med 148:1914–1918, 1988

Clarfield AM: The reversible dementias: do they reverse? Ann Intern Med 109:476–486, 1988

Gorbien MJ: Alcoholism in the elderly: the Sepulveda GRECC method. Geriatric Medicine Today 8:115–118, 1989

Hankin JR, Steinwachs DM, Regier DA, et al: Use of general medical care service by persons with mental disorders. Arch Gen Psychiatry 39:225–231, 1982

Hippocrates: Aphorisms, in Writings. Translated by Brock AJ. Franklin Center, PA, The Franklin Library, 1979, p 294

Hodkinson H: Non-specific presentation of illness. Br Med J 4:94–96, 1973

Koenig HG, Meador KG, Cohen HJ, et al: Depression in elderly hospitalized patients with medical illness. Arch Intern Med 148:1929–1936, 1988

Lamy PP: Prescribing for the Elderly. Littleton, CT, PSG Publishing, 1980

Lewis MA, Cretin S, Kane RL: The natural history of nursing home patients. Gerontologist 25:382–388, 1985

Lipowsky ZJ: Delirium in the elderly patient. N Engl J Med 320:578–586, 1989

Peters NL: Snipping the thread of life: antimuscarinic side effects of medications in the elderly. Arch Intern Med 149:2414–2420, 1989

Shamoian CA: Psychogeriatrics, in The Medical Clinics of North America: Symposium on Clinical Geriatric Medicine, Vol. 67. Edited by Samiy AH. Philadelphia, PA, WB Saunders, 1983, pp 361–378

Stewart RB, Caranasos GJ: Medication compliance in the elderly, in The Medical Clinics of North America: Geriatric Medicine: A Problem Oriented Approach, Vol 73. Edited by Bender BS, Caranasos GJ. Philadelphia, PA, WB Saunders, 1983, pp 1551–1563

Wilson LA, Lawson IR, Bross W: Multiple disorders in the elderly: a clinical and statistical study. Lancet 2:841–843, 1962

Chapter Nine

CANCER IN THE ELDERLY: PSYCHIATRIC ISSUES AND TREATMENT

Hindi T. Mermelstein, M.D., Jamie S. Ostroff, Ph.D., and Mary Jane Massie, M.D.

Older individuals with cancer constitute a special patient population growing in both numbers and interest to the medical and psychiatric communities. People over the age of 65 years comprise 11% of the population but account for 50% of the cancer cases in the United States. The incidence of neoplastic disease rises with increasing age. Each of the common cancers in the elderly population (e.g., lung, colorectal and esophagus, skin, prostate, breast, ovarian and uterine, non-Hodgkin's lymphoma, and chronic lymphocytic leukemia) has its own characteristics, course, treatment, and cure rates, but overall cancer mortality increases with age (Crawford and Cohen 1987) and is now the second leading cause of death among elderly people.

In recent years, the increased efficacy of treatment has translated into increased survival time for many oncology patients, including elderly ones. Recent work indicates that older patients tolerate the physical side effects (Begg and Carbone 1983) and psychological distress of chemotherapy as well as their younger counterparts (Ganz et al. 1985; Nerenz et al. 1986). Older patients also tolerate major cancer surgery, although they have increased rates of perioperative complications secondary to concurrent medical conditions (Crawford and Cohen 1987; Linn 1989). As a result of these findings, a high percentage of older patients are treated aggressively with good rates of remission and cure.

Most patients describe cancer as a catastrophic event. For the older person, this burden must be added to those of aging and of the socially isolating stigma of the disease itself. These psychosocial issues exacerbate the difficulties already present for the cancer patient. Psychiatric treatment can help some oncology patients deal with the changes in themselves and their world as the illness and its consequences unfold.

The Psychosocial Collaborative Oncology Group studied over 200 hospitalized and ambulatory adult patients of all ages, including elderly patients, at three different cancer centers. They found that over half (53%) were coping well (Derogatis et al. 1983). The remainder (47%) had a psychiatric disorder as diagnosed by DSM-III (American Psychiatric Association 1980) criteria. Most of the diagnoses (32% of the total population studied) were adjustment disorders with depression, anxiety, or both. Major depression accounted for 6% of the group, organic disorders for 4%, and premorbid personality and anxiety states for another 5%. When the prevalence of psychiatric disorders was studied specifically in older age groups, depression was found to be slightly more prevalent and adjustment disorders slightly less so than in younger age groups (Massie and Holland 1987a). Additionally, the group found a marked increase in the number of elderly patients diagnosed with delirium (Levine et al. 1978).

In this chapter, we will briefly outline the psychiatric issues found in elderly cancer patients and some of the interventions that are helpful with this special population. This chapter is organized according to the phases in the course of a cancer illness: time of diagnosis, active treatment, palliation, terminal illness, and survivorhood.

PSYCHOLOGICAL ISSUES SURROUNDING DIAGNOSIS

Cancer Detection/Delay in Diagnosis

Regardless of age, the best predictor of cancer survival remains early detection and treatment. Regular Pap smears, breast examinations, and other cancer screening tests can detect tumors at early, curable stages. The older a woman is, however, the less likely she is to have received these checkups on a regular basis or to have ever had them at all (Celantano 1989; Foster and Costanza 1984; Grover et al. 1989; List 1987).

Holland (1989) reviewed studies of patient delay in seeking medical consultation and reported that 75% of individuals postpone the consultation for at least one month after they find a suspicious symptom. Lower educational status and socioeconomic class, pessimism and fatalism about cancer, fear of being placed in a dependent role, and a poor doctor-patient relationship are factors contributing to this delay in all groups of patients studied (Holland 1989). These factors may play an even stronger role with the older patient inasmuch as elderly persons as a group delay seeking treatment longer than younger persons. Many older people still believe that a diagnosis of cancer is a death sentence and that the treatment is worse than the disease, so why go to the doctor (Wilson et al. 1984)? Older patients either may not have a doctor or may not feel comfortable in their relationship with their physician. This perception of nonalliance, when coupled with feelings of social isolation and worries about the financial burden of medical care, contributes to the reluctance to seek medical consultation (Holland and Massie 1987; Snider 1980). Physicians, as well as their older patients, often dismiss symptoms as part of "old age" or presume the symptoms are secondary to the patients' other medical conditions (Levkoff et al. 1988; Samiy 1983). Unfortunately, the prolonged delay in diagnosis increases the likelihood that the tumor will be at an advanced stage when it is discovered, with a consequently poor outcome for the patient.

Reaction to Diagnosis

The word *cancer* evokes fears of pain, suffering, and death in most people. They react to the diagnosis as they would to other extreme stressors, with shock, denial, anger, emotional lability, and anxiety. These responses can interfere with sleep, concentration, and participation in one's usual interests (Massie and Holland 1988; Weissman and Worden 1976–1977). These grieflike symptoms are befitting reactions to the threat of the loss of health, life roles, and the relationship with important objects through the possible loss of life itself. For the majority of patients, this intense emotional diathesis abates within a week or two. The best treatment for this normal response is emotional support usually provided by the oncologist or primary care physician (Massie and Holland 1987b). However, in cases where the outpouring of feelings is extreme or prolonged or actually interferes with the patient receiving medical care, psychiatric intervention can be effective. In spite of the initial discomfort some elderly individuals have with the idea of seeing a psychiatrist and of being labeled "crazy" as well as sick and old, psychiatric support and treatment can be most helpful.

PSYCHIATRIC ISSUES IN ACTIVE TREATMENT

Active treatment of the cancer, which is defined as the length of time following the diagnosis through the entire period of therapy itself, is a universally stressful period. During this phase, the psychiatrist is likely to see patients with depression, adjustment disorders, anxiety, and the organic mental syndromes.

Several groups have reported that older patients adapt better to illness than younger patients. This was found to be true regardless of the presence of other concurrent, chronic, disabling diseases (Cassileth et al. 1984) or of lower socioeconomic status (Maisiak et al. 1983). Ganz and colleagues (1985) studied the psychosocial problems of 240 male cancer patients matched for functional status, and they compared those over the age of 65 with those under 65. These investigators found that those patients over 65 adapted better to cancer treatment. This may represent prior acclimation to the health care system or the general trend for elderly patients to use more mature coping skills (McCrae 1982).

Adjustment Disorders and Major Depression

As noted earlier, in cancer patients of any age, adjustment disorders and depression are the most commonly diagnosed psychiatric illnesses. Many of the risk factors that predispose to these syndromes, including social isolation, a history of recent object losses, pessimism, dysphoria, socioeconomic pressures, and having a more advanced stage of disease, are more prevalent in elderly patients (Flaherty et al. 1983; Holland and Massie 1987; Kennedy et al. 1989). Adjustment disorders in the cancer patient often have associated features of depression and/or anxiety.

It is often presumed that anyone with cancer would, and perhaps even should, be depressed. This attitude contributes to an underdiagnosing of depression, which, if left untreated, leads to considerable morbidity for patients in terms of emotional distress, diminished social skills, and a decrease in their ability to participate in their own health care (Grassi et al. 1989; Harris et al. 1988; Klerman 1989). Another problem encountered in diagnosing depression in this population is uncertainty about just what diagnostic criteria to employ. Most clinical descriptions and many rating scales for depression include disturbances in sleep, appetite, and concentration, which can occur in cancer patients solely as a result of their medical condition. Thus, the presence of cancer may negate the usefulness of diagnostic scales such as the Zung and neuroendocrine measures such as the dexamethasone stimulation test, which have been clinically validated in older adults without cancer (Blazer 1989; Evans et al. 1986). Endicott (1984) proposed substituting social withdrawal, brooding or self-pity, the presence or absence of tearfulness, and an inability to be cheered up for the somatic symptoms of change in appetite or weight, change in sleep, psychomotor retardation or agitation, and decreased concentration. Rapp and Vrana (1989) found these substituted criteria to be sensitive and specific for the diagnosis of depression in their study of 150 elderly medically ill patients. Based on our clinical experience at Memorial Hospital, we concur that persistent dysphoria, feelings of helplessness, loss of self-esteem, feelings of worthlessness, and wishes to die are good diagnostic indicators for depression.

The task of the psychiatric consultant is complicated by the need to identify specific medical conditions or individual medications that may contribute to the onset or the intensity of the mood disorder. This is even more crucial in elderly patients because 50% have two or more concurrent illnesses and often take multiple medications that affect the central nervous system (CNS) (Wood et al. 1988). In addition, the consultant is often called upon to differentiate the apathy of early dementia from the blunting of affect, decrease in concentration, and other signs of pseudodementia observed in depression (Grossberg and Nakra 1988; Reynolds et al. 1988). Many of the commonly used chemotherapeutic agents, including corticosteroids (prednisone and dexamethasone), vinblastine, vincristine, and procarbazine, cause mood changes (Patchell and Posner 1985). Pain can also lead to anxiety, depressive symptoms, sleep disruptions, and personality disturbances. In the presence of even moderate pain, the definitive diagnosis of depression should be deferred until the pain has been adequately controlled (Breitbart 1989a).

Elderly individuals along with cancer patients of all ages suffer from fears of object loss, disability, dependency, and death (Goldberg and Cullen 1986; Silberfarb and Greer 1982). These underlying psychodynamic issues, which are important concerns in the instances of depression, dysphoria, and anxiety seen in aged persons (Berezin and Cath 1965; Blum and Tross 1980; Hiatt 1971; Nemiroff and Colarusso 1985), are usually intensified in the elderly cancer patient.

Modalities of Treatment

Supportive therapy. The most common type of psychotherapeutic intervention in the acute care of the cancer patient is supportive therapy based on the crisis intervention model (Capone et al. 1979; Massie et al. 1989). The very existence of a definitive diagnosis of cancer underscores the reality for the patient of a limited future. For the older cancer patient, this may provide strong motivational im-

New Techniques in the Psychotherapy of Older Patients

petus for psychotherapy (Myers 1984). King's (1980) concept of this being the last chance in one's life to modify long-standing emotional problems encourages some older cancer patients to seek intensive, exploratory psychotherapy after the acute crisis has been resolved. Vachon (1987) discussed the unresolved grief often seen in these patients while Rennecker (1957) reviewed the countertransference problems that arise in the course of therapy. The duration of therapy with these patients must remain flexible, and the therapist must recognize that a clear-cut termination may not be feasible because the therapist has become a "real" object for the patient. Active follow-up of patients after discharge from the hospital reinforces the idea of the therapist's availability and the recognition that psychosocial distress is an expected part of the cancer experience that can be treated.

The initial evaluation of such patients should include a baseline mental status examination, an assessment of the meaning of the illness to the individual within the context of previous experience with sickness, a history of the handling of prior stressful situations, and an assessment of the emotional support systems available to the patients (Lipowski 1970; Viederman 1983). The goals of supportive treatment include enabling patients to use their resources, returning them to their previous level of functioning, and helping them to develop better coping skills.

The therapist can help patients adjust to the changes within their bodies and themselves and to their heightened dependency needs while at the same time enabling the patients to preserve their sense of self-esteem. At times of acute changes in body image, such as after an operation or in the period of acute hair loss following chemotherapy, it is important for patients to continue to perceive themselves as whole persons. To help accomplish this aim, the therapist may encourage and reinforce feelings within the patient of being an involved, active member of the treatment team, both in the hospital and after discharge. Another function for the therapist is as patient advocate and supporter. This role is more important with elderly individuals who may have fewer external supports and may also fear becoming dependent on their children. Forester et al. (1985) found that patients who were in psychotherapy during their course of radiation had significantly less emotional distress and fewer physical complaints. With patients who felt isolated and disconnected from their oncologists, the bridging role played by the psychotherapist allowed the individual to feel supported.

Behavior therapy. Behavior therapy is a useful adjuvant in the treatment of depressive symptomatology in the older cancer patient.

148

Interventions can be tailored to fit the specific symptoms as well as the cognitive capacity of the individual patient. Positive reinforcement, usually in the form of enhanced social contacts, can increase the patient's constructive activities and personal hygiene. Improvement in activity level and in personal autonomy often translates directly into feelings of improved mood. Baltes (1988) reported that dependent self-care behaviors such as not attempting to feed oneself generally elicit attention (both positive and negative) and assistance from staff whereas independent self-care behaviors are virtually ignored. Therefore, encouraging the medical staff and family members to promote independent behavior is helpful.

Group therapy can enhance the effectiveness of behavioral treatment because of the built-in supportive social milieu, which may be lacking for many elderly patients. Recent work has also shown the utility of cognitive-behavioral therapies for depression in these patients (Gallagher and Thompson 1981; Patterson and Moon 1985). Adapting these strategies to the oncological setting and exploring patients' beliefs about their cancer or its treatment may reveal irrational or unhelpful thoughts that lead to feelings of helplessness and hopelessness. Correcting these depression-eliciting thoughts may be an effective therapeutic intervention.

Psychopharmacological agents. Antidepressant medication may alleviate depressed affect, irritability, emotional lability, and social withdrawal. Small (1989) reviewed the treatment of elderly depressed patients with medical illnesses. Tricyclic antidepressants are the drugs most often used in older patients with cancer. Nortriptyline causes the least orthostatic hypotension and is therefore best tolerated by geriatric patients (Roose and Glassman 1989). Medications with sedative properties, such as amitriptyline and doxepin, help alleviate the insomnia in these patients. Amitriptyline, imipramine, and doxepin, in addition to their antidepressant and sedative activity, also reduce pain and potentiate the narcotic analgesics (Massie and Holland 1984). Side effects from this group of medications include cardiac arrhythmias, anticholinergic-mediated delirium (Jefferson 1989; Meyers and Meital 1983), urinary retention, constipation, and dry mouth. These side effects are problematic for oncology patients with prostatic hypertrophy, those at risk for mechanical bowel obstruction, and those with stomatitis from chemotherapy or radiotherapy. Desipramine, the tricyclic with the least anticholinergic and epileptogenic properties, may be a good choice in patients at risk for these side effects or for seizures (Markowitz and Brown 1987). Several of the tricyclics are available in intramuscular (im), oral (po), and rectal

149

suppository form for patients who are unable to take oral medications or who cannot receive injections because of low platelet counts.

Before tricyclics are started, an electrocardiogram should be obtained. In older patients with cancer, all psychotropics are started at low doses. For example, a starting nortriptyline dose of 25 mg po qhs is raised very slowly by 25 mg po every 5–7 days. For as yet unclear reasons, doses as low as 30–40 mg qd of nortriptyline may be effective for some cancer patients (Massie and Holland 1989). Drug levels can be monitored in those patients who develop side effects on small doses of medication. This may be especially important in elderly patients who have age-induced alterations in drug metabolism (Pollack and Perel 1989).

Patients who cannot tolerate the tricyclics should receive a trial with other agents. For instance, alprazolam is a benzodiazepine with some antidepressant as well as anxiolytic effects. It has no anticholinergic side effects, so it is well tolerated by elderly oncology patients (Pitts et al. 1983; Rickels et al. 1985). In our experience, it is most effective for mild depressions or adjustment disorders. Side effects include behavioral disinhibition in patients with mild cognitive problems, dysphoria, and a higher addictive potential than most drugs of this class. Starting doses are 0.25 mg bid to tid, and average daily doses are in the 4–6 mg qd range. Fluoxetine, a new agent without anticholinergic effects (Cooper 1988), has a half-life of greater than 2 weeks. This can be problematic for unstable patients whose medications change rapidly. The monoamine oxidase inhibitors (MAOIs) are safe in older patients (Georgotas et al. 1986); however, necessary food restrictions add an additional burden to the life of the already restricted cancer patient. Severe (even lethal) toxicity caused by the combination of MAOIs and narcotics (e.g., demerol) severely limits the utilization of these drugs in an oncology setting. For those patients who need lithium carbonate, careful attention needs to be paid to the patient's fluid and electrolyte balances. This is particularly important in the perioperative period. For patients with mild depression in addition to mild confusional states, thioridazine may be effective in doses as low as 10 mg po bid or tid.

In the elderly depressed patient, stimulant medications have been shown to be safe and effective (Fernandez et al. 1987; Katon and Raskind 1980). Methylphenidate can improve the patient's mood, appetite, and sense of well-being while at the same time decreasing fatigue and counteracting the sedative effects of narcotics. Most patients respond quickly to this medication. A frequent starting dose is 5–10 mg qd or bid. All doses are given in the morning or early afternoon so as not to interfere with the patient's sleep. Psychostimulants

150

can safely produce rapid and continuing relief of depressive symptoms in the medically ill geriatric patients in whom tricyclic antidepressants are contraindicated (Satel and Nelson 1989). The following case illustrates the merits of multimodal clinical interventions in the treatment of depression in the older cancer patient.

Case Example

A 67-year-old woman with stage III ovarian cancer was referred to psychiatry for depression. The patient stated that she and her husband had handled her illness well until one month ago, when the disease recurred. Since then she felt depressed, stopped going out with friends, had crying spells, and at times even felt too fatigued to get dressed. Her appetite diminished, and she began using temazepam nightly for sleep. She added that both she and her husband had lost parents and friends to cancer, and they felt unable to go through another cancer death. She exhibited no evidence of psychotic thinking, suicidal ideation, or cognitive dysfunction. The patient was seen in individual supportive psychotherapy, where the themes of her fear of loss of control in the context of her heightened dependency needs and physical debility were explored. In family sessions, the patient, her husband, and their children discussed the changes in their family roles and the anxieties and communication problems that resulted from the shift in intrafamily structure. She was also started on nortriptyline, 25 mg po qd, which was increased to 75 mg qhs. Her mood brightened, her interest in outside activities returned, and her sleep pattern improved. When she developed stomatitis from her chemotherapy, she was unable to tolerate the nortriptyline-induced dry mouth and was switched to fluoxetine, again with good result.

Suicide

In an article entitled "Is It Normal for Terminally Ill Patients to Desire Death?" Brown et al. (1986) reported that only 10 out of 44 patients studied wanted to die early. All 10 suffered from a clinical depressive disorder, which has been determined to be a major risk factor in suicide in the cancer patient (Breitbart 1989b).

The risk of suicide is increased in patients who are older, in those with prominent premorbid psychopathology, in those who have a personal or family history of suicidal behavior, and in those with poor psychosocial supports (Saunders and Valente 1988). Ancillary factors that add to the risk of suicide in cancer patients include delirium, advanced disease, head and neck tumors that are associated with disfigurement, and a history of substance abuse and poorly controlled pain. A common period for intensification of suicidal feelings is at the point of treatment failure, when the patient is told "nothing more can be done." The most important psychodynamic issue in suicidal behavior in cancer patients is the enormous loss of control these patients feel. Suicidal ideation is frequent although suicide attempts, per se, are not. Active suicidal ideation often represents a means for patients to maintain an illusory sense of control over their deaths, if not over their bodies or their lives.

The psychiatrist must assess the patients' level of intent, their inner and external control systems and supports, and the meaning of suicide for them. Many patients become less suicidal once the therapist acknowledges the legitimacy of the option and the normalcy of the patient's need to maintain a sense of control. The essential feature in the management of such individuals involves the reduction of pain, anxiety, and depression, with a consequent lessening of feelings of unnecessary desperation.

Anxiety and Insomnia

Anxiety and insomnia are frequent complaints of elderly patients. In cancer patients, acute anxiety occurs at times of illness-related stress—for example, while awaiting test results, before surgery and major procedures, and at the start of chemotherapy or radiotherapy. It usually responds to supportive interventions and sedation the night before major procedures and surgery. Multiple organic bases for anxiety in elderly cancer patients may be found. For example, individuals with respiratory distress or with cardiac disease often have anxiety that may be relieved by analgesics, oxygen cardiovasodilators, and the judicious addition of a mild sedative. Many medications, such as bronchodilators (theophylline) and corticosteroids, may cause anxiety and agitation even at therapeutic doses. Other organic causes of anxiety to be considered in the differential diagnosis include early delirium, alcohol and drug withdrawal, thyroid and endocrine disorders, pheochromocytomas, brain tumors (both primary and secondary), and carcinoid syndromes.

In cancer patients, almost all cases of chronic anxiety disorders (phobias and panic disorders) predate the cancer diagnosis. Problems such as needle phobias or claustrophobia may lead to delay in necessary medical examinations or in tests such as the magnetic resonance imaging scans. When test results are needed urgently, as is often the case in an oncological setting, mild sedation is suggested before such procedures are administered.

152

Modalities of Treatment

Relaxation techniques.   Relaxation training by means of progressive muscle relaxation, the use of mental imagery, or hypnosis is also helpful in reducing anxiety. These techniques are effective in distracting patients from anxiety-provoking thoughts and painful sensations, in reducing autonomic arousal, and in providing a sense of personal control. Most geriatric cancer patients can successfully learn to use relaxation techniques effectively. Clinicians should tailor the relaxation techniques according to the patient's presenting problem and coping style, and then instruct and demonstrate the relaxation procedures to the patient. It is often helpful to prepare an audiotape of the instructions to facilitate practice between therapy sessions.

Psychopharmacological agents.   When the anxious cancer patient needs medication in addition to supportive psychotherapy and behavioral interventions, the benzodiazepines are the drugs of choice. The short-acting benzodiazepines, such as lorazepam, do not have active metabolites that accumulate as do diazepam or chlorazepate. Lorazepam is well absorbed by the oral, intravenous (iv), and im routes and is not metabolized by the liver—both added benefits in the older, medically ill patient who often has age and/or disease-induced diminished hepatic function. Daily doses of lorazepam are small—in the 0.5–1 mg tid range. The most common side effects are drowsiness, confusion, and motor incoordination (Cutler and Narang 1984), which, if marked, may look like a dementia in the elderly patient. The side effects are dose dependent, and some tolerance to the drowsiness develops with continued use. Lorazepam's antiemetic properties are particularly useful in the oncological setting. Many patients who receive iv lorazepam as part of their antiemetic regimen are amnestic for part or all of their chemotherapy. Elderly patients, who are fearful that this memory loss is a symptom of senility, should be reassured that the amnesia is drug related and will only be temporary. Another risk of benzodiazepines is their synergism with other CNS depressants such as the narcotic analgesics, which may lead to inordinate depths of sedation and respiratory depression.

The antihistamines are sometimes used in patients with respiratory compromise, but they are not as effective as the benzodiazepines in achieving an anxiolytic or sedative effect. Antihistamines are strongly anticholinergic and can lead to delirium, which may contribute to the functional disability in the older patient (Miller et al. 1988; Rovner et al. 1988). Antipsychotics are reserved for the agitation of organic mental

153

syndromes. Buspirone, a nonbenzodiazepine, may benefit some patients with a generalized anxiety syndrome, but it is less effective in the acute hospital setting because there may be a lag of 2–3 weeks between the start of medication and the onset of antianxiety effects. Its most common side effects include headache, dizziness, and nausea (Sussman 1988).

Over 60% of the older population complain of insomnia because of the fragmentation of sleep that comes with normal aging. The disruptive effects of acute hospital care, poorly controlled pain, and intrusive illness-related thoughts intensify the problem. For acute care, the benzodiazepines are the drugs most commonly used. Triazolam has an ultrashort half-life, which makes it good for people with initial rather than middle or late insomnia. This medication can, however, cause rebound anxiety and memory problems the day after being used. Temazepam and flurazepam are also effective but can cause daytime sedation. For chronic insomnia reassurance, the options of environmental manipulation, behavior modification, and psychotherapeutic interventions should be tried before hypnotics are considered (Moran et al. 1988).

Case Example
A 69-year-old man with lung cancer and a recent myocardial infarction was referred to psychiatry for treatment of anxiety and depression. He described himself as "jittery." Respiratory difficulty, ruminative thinking about his illness, and anxiety symptoms interfered with his sleep. He was mildly dysphoric, irritable, anxious, and tremulous. Although generally oriented, he had decreased concentration and a diminished attention span. When his theophylline level was lowered from borderline-toxic to normal range, his tremor disappeared. There was no change in his subjective sense of agitation, however, so alprazolam was prescribed. His anxiety decreased, but he remained depressed and irritable and felt too fatigued to participate in a rehabilitation program. Given his underlying cardiac disease, he could not be switched to a tricyclic antidepressant, and the dose of alprazolam could not be increased because of concomitant respiratory compromise. Consequently, methylphenidate was added. The patient's appetite, energy level, and involvement in physical therapy improved. He and his family were amenable to supportive psychotherapy, where the need for the family members to continue to communicate and not turn away from one another in their anger and anxiety about his illness was stressed. Psychiatric treatment was continued on an outpatient basis after discharge from the hospital.

Delirium

Delirium occurs frequently in the cancer patient. Twenty percent of all consultation requests at Memorial Hospital are for management of delirium. The incidence of delirium rises to 75% of terminally ill cancer patients (Massie et al. 1983). Delirium is a global disturbance of attention, cognition, psychomotor activity, and the sleep-wake cycle. The onset may be sudden or gradual, and the symptoms fluctuate over the course of the day and intensify at night (sundowning). Early symptoms such as irritability, withdrawal, restlessness, and sleep disturbance are often missed or misdiagnosed by the medical staff. Levine and colleagues (1978) found that many older patients who were referred for treatment of depression actually suffered from a delirium. Patients may be too frightened and embarrassed to report such symptoms to their physicians. As the syndrome progresses, affective lability and suspiciousness or paranoia are common. Perceptual disturbances and poorly formed hallucinations occur in 40–50% of elderly delirious patients (Lipowski 1989).

The risk of delirium is increased in patients who are over 65 and have preexisting cerebral damage and a history of alcohol abuse. Delirium in cancer patients is due both to the direct effects of the cancer on the CNS and to the indirect CNS complications of the disease and/or the treatment, including changes in electrolyte and fluid balance, medications, sepsis, nutritional status, vascular complications, and hormone-secreting tumors (Patchell and Posner 1985; Silberfarb and Oxman 1988). Medications that frequently cause delirium in the older oncology patient are narcotics, corticosteroids, psychotropics, and, less frequently, chemotherapeutic agents. In the setting of these risk factors and metabolic derangements, delirium is often precipitated by sleep deprivation, sensory overload, and immobilization (Lipowski 1989).

Once delirium is suspected, a careful review of the patient's medical and mental status and laboratory values is indicated. Sometimes, the symptoms must be treated while the search for the etiology is still underway.

Modalities of Treatment

Supportive measures. The management of delirium includes reassurance, monitoring, environmental manipulation, and medication. Patients benefit from short, repeated visits with known family members who can reassure and reorient them. Fortunately, most patients cannot recall the delirious period. Some may remember it as a frightening experience and may need help integrating it once the acute episode remits. Family and friends are often worried that their loved one is losing his or her mind during a delirious episode.

155

The consultant should carefully educate and reassure the family about the cause, probable course, and expected resolution of the delirium. Ideally, there should be continuity of nursing care from shift to shift. When agitation and confusion are severe, or when the patient is actively hallucinating, 24-hour companions are needed to prevent the patient from harming self and others. Delirious patients may have suicidal ideation secondary to their terror and confused thinking. This, combined with the poor impulse control and impaired judgment that are an integral part of delirium, puts the patient at risk for accidental self-injury.

Environmental manipulation. Environmental manipulation includes decreasing sensory overload. Patients may benefit from a night-light in their room, calendars, and other methods to limit disorientation from loss of visual cues. Severe delirium is one of the few psychiatric indications for a single-bed room in a medical setting.

Psychopharmacological agents. Pharmacological intervention usually consists of antipsychotic medication, preferably with a high-potency drug such as haloperidol in doses of 0.25–0.5 mg po, im, or iv q 4–6 hours. Haloperidol can improve the patient's cognitive state without the ancillary sedation and the concomitant risk of hypotension often seen with the phenothiazines or benzodiazepines, especially when they are administered parenterally. Elderly patients are at risk for extrapyramidal side effects, which respond to the judicious use of antiparkinsonian agents such as benztropine (Salzman 1987). In patients with poorly controlled seizures, molindone is the antipsychotic of choice.

Case Example

A 79-year-old man with advanced prostatic cancer was admitted to Memorial Hospital for radiation of cervical spine metastases. When he demanded to leave the hospital to see his mother to calm his restlessness, he was referred for psychiatric consultation. He was oriented as to time, place, and person but did not know how long he had been hospitalized. He was aware of having cancer but did not know why he was scheduled for radiation treatment. He complained of strange odors and noises that kept him up at night but that did not bother him during the day. As his condition worsened, there was a great fluctuation in his mental status. At times he was coherent, and yet several hours later he would be screaming or actively hallucinating. Medications included oxycodone and lorazepam. According to the nurses' notes, his oral intake was poor and he was dehydrated and hyponatremic.

The patient's delirium was caused by a confluence of multiple factors,

156

so a number of different interventions were utilized. His fluid and sodium levels were corrected, the lorazepam was tapered, and the narcotic dosage was lowered. Because of his agitation and paranoia, he was moved to a private room and a 24-hour companion was ordered. His wife was terrified that he had gone "crazy," and her anxiety was alleviated by frequent reassurances from the psychiatrist. The patient was started on haloperidol 0.5 mg bid and 1 mg qhs plus prn doses. A week later, with his delirium completely resolved, the episode only remained in his memory in a hazy manner.

Other Psychiatric Disorders

In elderly cancer patients, the entire spectrum of psychiatric disorders may be seen. Many older patients suffer from paranoid ideation secondary to social isolation, sensory loss, and diminished communication skills (Stoudemire and Riether 1987). In cases of late onset delusional states, especially in the medically ill patient, there should be an aggressive search for an underlying and perhaps reversible etiology. For a review of the causes, characteristics, and treatment of other psychiatric disorders in elderly patients, interested readers should refer to Busse and Blazer (1989).

Compliance With Treatment

The treatment of cancer has become a prolonged process, with multiple hospitalizations, doctor appointments, care by different medical personnel, and the need for repeated follow-up tests and procedures. Good compliance with treatment recommendations is essential for optimal therapeutic results. Maisiak and colleagues (1983) found that, due to a lack of faith in treatment and the confusion of the medical setting, older patients missed appointments more often than younger patients. The presence of a supportive person to help the patient get the needed services, the use of repeated explanations of the goals of treatment, and the amelioration of psychiatric disorders enhance the older patient's compliance with arduous treatment regimens (Massie and Holland 1989). Behavioral rehearsal is also effective in helping elderly cancer patients and their family caregivers gain a sense of mastery and comfort with self-care medical procedures. By reducing the anxiety and confusion associated with self-care procedures, accurate and consistent adherence to the treatment regimen is enhanced.

PSYCHIATRIC ISSUES IN PALLIATION

When the patient moves into the palliative period, the primary goal of treatment shifts to maximizing the patient's current functioning and comfort and all of the components encompassed under the rubric "quality of life." The primary psychiatric issue during this period is pain control.

Pain Control

Patients repeatedly inform us that they are not as afraid of death as they are of suffering during the dying process. Patients in pain have higher rates of anxiety, depression, hostility, and other psychiatric symptoms that may be alleviated by pain relief. In the presence of pain, the premorbid personality structure cannot be accurately determined. Uncontrolled pain is a major risk factor for suicidal behavior in the cancer patient.

In the last few years, much has been learned about pain and about ways to deal with the narcotic side effects (Foley 1989) as well as other physical symptoms of the older oncology patient during the palliative phase (Cobbs and Lynn 1989). Pain is multidetermined and should be treated with a multimodal approach. The psychiatric interventions in pain management are pharmacotherapy, psychotherapy, education, relaxation training, visual imagery, and group therapy (Breitbart 1989a).

In the terminal phases of cancer, good pain control is essential. The older patient is very susceptible to opiate-induced delirium. Though antipsychotics may decrease paranoia and improve concentration, the symptoms of the delirium may be only partially treatable. In cases in which a choice of comfort versus coherence is necessary, the psychiatrist's role as patient advocate is important.

Case Example

A 70-year-old man with end-stage sarcoma, admitted to Memorial Hospital for pain control, was referred to psychiatry after he repeatedly stated he wanted to die. He told the consultant his pain was so severe that he was unable to eat or sleep, and he wished that he were dead. He accused the staff of torturing him by decreasing his pain medication. He had visual and auditory hallucinations. He was oriented to person but not to time or place. This confusional state persisted despite correction of his electrolyte disturbance and decrease in his narcotic medication. Because of his terminal status, an aggressive search for nonopiate, nonelectrolyte-related etiologies of his delirium was not performed.

The psychiatric consultant felt that this patient's dose of narcotics should be titrated according to the patient's level of pain and not his level of delirium. With the addition of haloperidol, the patient's paranoia and belligerence lessened although he continued to hallucinate. The patient decided to continue the opiates and stated, "I'll learn to live with my old buddies popping in and out of my room. I can't live with the pain." His wife, who herself had a heart condition, originally felt unable to care for him at home. When his paranoia decreased and health care at home was arranged, he was discharged there, where he remained until his death.

PSYCHIATRIC ISSUES IN THE TERMINAL PHASE

As the patient moves into the final stage of illness, some problems such as pain may continue to intensify. The main themes, however, are dying, grief, and bereavement.

Death and Dying

Just as cancer and aging have different meanings for each person, so too are our fantasies and concepts of death individualized (Bibring 1966). Commonality of concerns about death revolve around fears of the unknown, abandonment, loss from and to others, and loss of self-control (Pattison 1967), or, in more global Kohutian terms, around fears of self-fragmentation and loss of self-cohesion (Tasman 1982).

Dying patients all share an underlying fear of abandonment. When patients, even early in the course of their disease, talk about dying, they want to know not only what can be done to alleviate suffering but also who will be there with them at the point of their demise. In the current medical setting, some of these concerns are reality based. The anxiety that medical personnel experience secondary to their inability to cure patients may cause them to distance themselves emotionally from these patients during terminal phases (Spikes and Holland 1975). For the family, death from cancer differs from death from many other illnesses inasmuch as the death is expected so anticipatory grief is allowed to take place. Intense grief reactions for family members occur at crisis points in the illness much as they do for the patients themselves (Koocher 1986; Schmale 1976). As the course of cancer becomes a chronic one with repeated crises and remissions, the family may have completed their grief work and emotionally detached themselves from the dying member too early. When patients are dying and need family support and comfort most, they may have already been emotionally abandoned (Fulton and Fulton 1971).

159

Specific psychiatric interventions toward the patients in this period are hard to outline because this is the time when the greatest therapeutic latitude and flexibility are needed. All of us who have worked with dying patients know that sometimes contact means physical touching, and sessions may consist of literal hand-holding. Eissler (1955) spoke of the relationship between the psychiatrist and the dying patient as the special gift situation. In all age groups, the psychiatrist gives to the dying patient by "being there," but, as noted previously, this has added importance for older patients.

Bereavement

Grief is the normal and necessary process of integrating the loss of an emotionally bound person and returning to life. In the bereavement period, there is increased mortality and morbidity, most markedly for the older male widower (Helsing and Szklo 1981). Since cancer death is generally expected, there is an opportunity to help the family prepare for the patient's death. Pasnau and colleagues (1987) have outlined a guide for physicians vis-à-vis the family prior to, at the time of, and after the identified patient's death. Follow-up phone contact or visits reinforce the concept of the physician's availability and continued support during the stressful mourning and bereavement period.

PSYCHOLOGICAL ISSUES DURING SURVIVORHOOD

Recent advances in oncology have led to improved likelihood for long-term disease-free survival. There has been a concomitant shift in the focus of psychosocial issues. In the past, the primary psychosocial themes evolved around death and dying. Now, it is also important to emphasize the patients' posttreatment quality of life as they reenter vocational, familial, and friendship networks (Tross and Holland 1989). Cancer patients are extremely happy to complete their treatment successfully; however, they may also feel frightened by the loss of close medical support from their treatment team and overwhelmed by the task of integrating precancer interests and activities with their cancer-related experiences and limitations.

Much attention has been given to the late medical effects of childhood cancer survivors. Antineoplastic therapy can adversely affect virtually all major body systems (Byrd 1985; Li 1977; Meadows and Hobbie 1986; Thompson et al. 1987). A recent review by Loescher and her colleagues (1989) provides an overview of the long-term physiological effects found in young adult cancer survivors. To date, no studies have specifically examined the medical sequelae of older cancer patients. Elderly survivors may not have the same long-term effects as pediatric and young adult cancer survivors.

Several studies have documented numerous psychosocial sequelae experienced by cancer survivors. Most notable among these are fear of recurrence, uncertainty about the future, heightened anxiety and depression, a sense of personal inadequacy, and a diminished sense of personal control (Fobair et al. 1986; Koocher and O'Malley 1981; Welch-McCaffrey et al. 1989). These feelings are not universal, however, and do not generally reach the magnitude of psychiatric illness (Lesko et al. 1986). Happily, even given these concerns and uncertainties, most cancer survivors experience good posttreatment adjustment (Schmale et al. 1983; Shanfield 1980). The amount of time since treatment completion is inversely related to the degree of psychological distress, with the period immediately following treatment completion representing a peak time of psychological vulnerability (Cella and Tross 1986). There have been no studies specifically examining the psychosocial sequelae experienced by elderly cancer survivors, and research in this area is sorely needed.

Finally, cancer survivors are faced with the task of reentering their social, family, and vocational roles (Tross and Holland 1989). Decreased physical stamina and heightened psychological distress can impede progress in this area. During active treatment, daily life for most cancer patients and their families evolves around the patients' disease and its treatment. Following successful treatment, patients and their families must resume developmentally appropriate tasks. Relationships with family and friends are often altered by cancer (Rait and Lederberg 1989). In contrast to the intense social support seen during active treatment, some cancer survivors experience posttreatment social isolation as well-intentioned family and friends avoid discussions of sensitive issues. While some cancer survivors may prefer to "selectively deny" or minimize the impact of cancer on their lives, others experience ongoing discussions of their cancer-related concerns as supportive and validating. In addition, some cancer survivors are afraid of burdening others with "posttreatment but cured" complaints and isolate themselves from social support systems.

Most cancer patients are able to cope with the stresses of survivorhood. Reassurances about the normalcy of their ambivalence enhance adjustment. However, for survivors with pathologically intense or persistent psychological distress, individual psychotherapy is warranted. There are a growing number of support groups geared toward the specific needs of cancer survivors. The American Cancer Society is a good community resource for mental health professionals and their patients.

Family therapy may also be helpful in reorganizing daily life around nonillness concerns and in renegotiating family roles and communication patterns that may have been altered during active treatment.

Case Example

One year after resection of a lung tumor, an 87-year-old woman was referred to psychiatry for evaluation and treatment of depression. The patient complained that before her illness she had been socially active, but since the surgery she had experienced mild shortness of breath and was unable to resume her usual activities. She felt overwhelmed by the realization that her remaining life span was limited, and she was constantly worried about the fate of her 22-year-old granddaughter (whom she had custody of) after she died. When a physical examination revealed no sign of recurrence of her cancer, the patient was referred for psychiatric consultation. On mental status examination her mood was dysphoric, without the hopelessness, guilty ruminations, or suicidal ideation of a severe major depressive episode. A diagnosis of adjustment disorder was made, and brief supportive psychotherapy was begun.

During the 2 months of this therapy, unresolved feelings of grief emerged as the major treatment issue. In the year or two before her cancer had been diagnosed, the patient had experienced multiple losses, including the death of her husband. These losses had prevented her from grieving for her own lost health. Through therapy, which helped her to review her life and her recent losses and got her to recognize the roles she continued to play, the patient was able to express her feelings of grief more adequately and to reconstitute more of her normal personality. She began to see herself as the same valuable woman she had always been, although with somewhat altered capabilities, and she no longer equated her disability with feelings of total invalidism or of living death.

Another obstacle to her coming to terms with her limited life span was the need she felt to be available to her granddaughter forever in order to compensate for her own daughter's having abandoned the child. Through exploration of her relationship with her grandchild, she was able to recognize that her granddaughter was a young adult and not a totally dependent child. The patient improved in brief therapy, became more outgoing, and even joined the local senior citizens club. However, both she and the consultant felt that there was more work to do to help her better understand some of these issues. She was consequently referred for long-term exploratory, psychodynamically oriented psychotherapy and is doing well.

SUMMARY AND FUTURE DIRECTIONS

In this chapter, we have outlined the common psychiatric problems and interventions in the older patient with cancer. The assault of cancer affects many systems and spheres in the patient's life, and the best treatment strategies are multidisciplinary ones. Most older patients have several chronic conditions, and rehabilitation services such as physical and occupational therapy may play a crucial role in optimizing patients' residual functioning and independence (MacVicar and Winningham 1986). The psychiatrist's role is to assess the patient's needs and to refer for and, at times, coordinate this multisystem treatment to maximize the patient's quality of life.

Case Example
A 79-year-old woman with pancreatic cancer was referred to psychiatry for noncompliance with treatment. She complained of poor balance and difficulty walking. She was organically impaired, with poor judgment and mild paranoia. Her previous medical history was unavailable, and it was unclear if there was dementia underlying the delirium that was present. With low doses of haloperidol and frequent visits by one nurse whom she began to trust, her paranoia lessened, her concentration and judgment improved, and she was able to cooperate with her care. Unfortunately, although she was too ill to care for herself, she lived alone and refused direct transfer to a hospice: "I'm not a package at Parcel Post. You just don't send me from one place to another." She wanted to go home for a week to settle her affairs first. Psychiatry, physical and occupational therapy, nursing, patient representatives, social work, and discharge planning worked together with this patient to maximize her self-care abilities and find her the considerable added support she needed at home. She got her wish and was home for 3 weeks before her final admission to a terminal care facility.

Recommendations for Future Research

A thorough review of the literature reveals a relative absence of empirical studies examining the psychosocial adjustment of older cancer patients.

Further clarification of the incidence, nature, and risk factors associated with psychiatric disorder among older cancer patients is needed to develop and refine prevention and rehabilitation efforts geared toward the maintenance of psychological health. Clinicians need to have a better understanding of how older cancer patients cope with the multitude of stressors inherent in cancer. It is premature to assume that the findings of research in psychooncology, which is generally based on younger samples of cancer patients, are applicable to the specific psychiatric symptomatology manifested by older cancer patients.

Prospective studies of older patients with various diagnoses and treatment regimens must be conducted. Longitudinal studies will allow researchers to observe when, during the course of cancer treatment, older patients experience psychological dysfunction. Finally, research that assesses multidimensional indexes of sociodemographic, medical, and psychological factors will help us identify factors predictive of optimal adjustment of older adult cancer patients.

As we learn more, we can better help our elderly cancer patients deal with the short- and long-term psychosocial consequences of their battle against the catastrophe of cancer.

REFERENCES

American Psychiatric Association: Diagnostic and Statistical Manual of Mental Disorders, 3rd Edition. Washington, DC, American Psychiatric Association, 1980

Baltes M: The etiology and maintenance of dependency in the elderly: three phases of operant research. Behavior Therapy 19:301–319, 1988

Begg C, Carbone P: Clinical trials and drug toxicity in the elderly: the experience of the Eastern Cooperative Oncology Group. Cancer 52:1986–1992, 1983

Berezin M, Cath S: Geriatric Psychiatry: Grief, Loss, and Emotional Disorders in the Aging Process. New York, International Universities Press, 1965

Bibring G: Old age: its liabilities and its assets: a psychological discourse, in Psychoanalysis: A General Psychology. Edited by Lowenstein R. New York, International Universities Press, 1966, pp 253–271

Blazer D: Depression in the elderly. N Engl J Med 320:164–166, 1989

Blum J, Tross S: Psychodynamic treatment of the elderly: a review of issues in theory and practice. Ann Rev Gerontol Geriatr 1:204–234, 1980

Breitbart W: Psychiatric management of cancer pain. Cancer 63:2336–2342, 1989a

Breitbart W: Suicide, in Handbook of Psychooncology: Psychological Care of the Patient With Cancer. Edited by Holland J, Rowland J. New York, Oxford University Press, 1989b, pp 291–300

Brown J, Henteloff P, Barakat S, et al: Is it normal for terminally ill patients to desire death? Am J Psychiatry 143:208–211, 1986

Busse E, Blazer D (eds): Geriatric Psychiatry. Washington, DC, American Psychiatric Press, 1989

Byrd R: Late effects of treatment of cancer in children. Pediatr Clin North Am 32:835–857, 1985

Capone M, Westie K, Chitwood J, et al: Crisis intervention: a functional model for hospitalized cancer patients. Am J Orthopsychiatry 49:598–607, 1979

Cassileth B, Lusk E, Strouse T, et al: Psychosocial status in chronic illness: a comparative analysis of six diagnostic groups. N Engl J Med 311:506–511, 1984

Celantano D: Prevention of cancer in the elderly, in Cancer and Aging: Progress in Research and Treatment. Edited by Zenser T, Cole R. New York, Springer, 1989, pp 187–209

Cella D, Tross S: Psychological adjustment to survival from Hodgkin's disease. J Consult Clin Psychol 54:616–622, 1986

Cobbs E, Lynn J: The care of the dying patient, in Principles of Geriatric Medicine and Gerontology. Edited by Hazzard W, Andres R, Bierman E, et al. New York, McGraw-Hill, 1989, pp 354–361

Cooper G: The safety of fluoxetine—an update. Br J Psychiatry 153 (suppl):77–86, 1988

Crawford J, Cohen H: Relationship of cancer and aging. Clin Geriatr Med 3:419–432, 1987

Cutler N, Narang P: Implications of dosing tricyclic antidepressants and benzodiazepines in geriatrics. Psychiatr Clin North Am 7:845–861, 1984

Derogatis L, Marrow G, Fetting J, et al: The prevalence of psychiatric disorders among cancer patients. JAMA 249:751–757, 1983

Eissler K: The Psychiatrist and the Dying Patient. New York, International Universities Press, 1955

Endicott J: Measurement of depression in patients with cancer. Cancer 53 (suppl):2243–2249, 1984

Evans D, McCartney D, Nemeroll C, et al: Depression in women treated for gynecological cancer: clinical and endocrine assessment. Am J Psychiatry 143:447–452, 1986

Fernandez F, Adams F, Holmes V, et al: Methylphenidate for depressive disorders in cancer patients. Psychosomatics 28:455–461, 1987

Flaherty J, Graviria M, Blach E, et al: The role of social support in the functioning of patients with unipolar depression. Am J Psychiatry 140:473–476, 1983

Fobair P, Hoppe R, Bloom J, et al: Psychosocial problems among survivors of Hodgkin's disease. J Clin Oncol 4:805–814, 1986

Foley K: Pain management in the elderly, in Principles of Geriatric Medicine and Gerontology. Edited by Hazzard W, Andres R, Bierman E, et al. New York, McGraw-Hill, 1989, pp 281–295

Forester B, Kornfield D, Fliess J: Psychotherapy during radiotherapy: effect on emotional and physical distress. Am J Psychiatry 142:22–27, 1985

Foster R, Costanza M: Breast self-examination practices and breast cancer survival. Cancer 53:999–1005, 1984

Fulton R, Fulton J: A psychosocial aspect of terminal care: anticipatory grief. Omega 2:91–100, 1971

Gallagher D, Thompson L: Depression in the Elderly: A Behavioral Treatment Manual. New York, Lexington, 1981

Ganz P, Schag MC, Heinrich R: The psychosocial impact of cancer on the elderly: a comparison with younger patients. J Am Geriatr Soc 3:429–435, 1985

Georgotas A, McCue R, Hapworth R, et al: Comparative efficacy and safety of MAOIs versus TCAs in treating depression in the elderly. Biol Psychiatry 21:1155–1166, 1986

Goldberg R, Cullen L: Depression in geriatric cancer patients: guide to assessment and treatment. Hospice Journal 2:79–98, 1986

Grassi L, Rosti G, Albieri C, et al: Depression and abnormal illness behavior in cancer patients. Gen Hosp Psychiatry 111:404–411, 1989

Grossberg G, Nakra R: The diagnostic dilemma of depressive pseudodementia, in Central Nervous System Disorders of Aging: Interventions and Research. Edited by Strong R. New York, Raven, 1988, pp 107–115

Grover S, Cook E, Adams J, et al: Delayed diagnosis of gynecological tumors in elderly women: relation to national medical practice patterns. Am J Med 86:151–157, 1989

Harris R, Mion L, Patterson M, et al: Severe illness in the older patients: the association between depressive disorders and functional dependency during the recovery phase. J Am Geriatr Soc 36:890–896, 1988

Helsing K, Szklo M: Mortality after bereavement. Am J Epidemiol 114:41–52, 1981

Hiatt H: Dynamic psychotherapy with the aging patient. Am J Psychother 25:591–600, 1971

Holland J: Fears and abnormal reactions to cancer in physically healthy individuals, in Handbook of Psychooncology: Psychological Care of the Patient With Cancer. Edited by Holland J, Rowland J. New York, Oxford University Press, 1989, pp 13–21

Holland J, Massie M: Psychosocial status of cancer in the elderly. Clin Geriatr Med 3:533–539, 1987

Jefferson J: Cardiovascular effects and toxicity of anxiolytics and antidepressants. J Clin Psychiatry 50:368–378, 1989

Katon W, Raskind M: Treatment of depression in the medically ill elderly with methylphenidate. Am J Psychiatry 137:963–965, 1980

Kennedy G, Kelman H, Thomas C, et al: Hierarchy of characteristics associated with depressive symptoms in an urban elderly sample. Am J Psychiatry 146:2220–2225, 1989

King P: The life cycle as indicated by the nature of the transference in the psychoanalysis of middle aged and elderly. Int J Psychoanal 61:153–160, 1980

Klerman G: Depressive disorders: further evidence for increased medical morbidity and impairment of social functioning. Arch Gen Psychiatry 46:856–858, 1989

Koocher G: Coping with a death from cancer. J Consult Clin Psychology 54:623–631, 1986

Koocher G, O'Malley J: The Damocles Syndrome: Psychosocial Consequences of Surviving Childhood Cancer. New York, McGraw-Hill, 1981

Lesko L, Mumma G, Mashberg D: Psychosocial functioning of adult acute leukemia survivors treated with bone marrow transplantation and standard chemotherapy. Proceedings of the Twenty-third Annual Meeting of the American Society of Clinical Oncology 5:1001, 1986

Levine P, Silberfarb P, Lipowski Z: Mental disorders in cancer patients: a study of 100 psychiatric referrals. Cancer 42:1385–1391, 1978

Levkoff S, Cleary P, Wette T, et al: Illness behavior in the aged: implications for clinicians. J Am Geriatr Soc 36:622–629, 1988

Li F: Follow-up of childhood cancer survivors. Cancer 84:1776–1778, 1977

Linn B: Surgical management of the elderly cancer patient, in Cancer and Aging: Progress in Research and Treatment. Edited by Zenser T, Cole R. New York, Springer, 1989, pp 210–221

Lipowski Z: Physical illness, the individual, and the coping processes. Psychiatry in Medicine 1:91–102, 1970

Lipowski Z: Delirium in the elderly patient. N Engl J Med 320:578–582, 1989

List N: Perspectives in cancer screening in the elderly. Clin Geriatr Med 3:435–445, 1987

Loescher L, Welch-McCaffrey D, Leigh S, et al: Surviving adult cancers, I: physiological effects. Ann Intern Med 111:411–432, 1989

MacVicar M, Winningham M: Promoting the functional capacity of cancer patients. The Cancer Bulletin 38:235–238, 1986

Maisiak R, Cams R, Lee E, et al: The psychological support status of elderly cancer outpatients. Prog Clin Biol Res 120:395–403, 1983

Markowitz J, Brown R: Seizures with neuroleptics and antidepressants. Gen Hosp Psychiatry 9:135–141, 1987

Massie MJ, Holland J: Diagnosis and treatment of depression in the cancer patient. J Clin Psychiatry 45:25–28, 1984

Massie MJ, Holland JC: The cancer patient with pain. Med Clin North Am 71:243–258, 1987a

Massie MJ, Holland JC: Consultation and liaison issues in cancer care. Psychiatr Med 5:343–359, 1987b

Massie MJ, Holland JC: Assessment and management of the cancer patient with depression. Adv Psychosom Med 1:1–12, 1988

Massie MJ, Holland JC: The older patient with cancer, in Handbook of Psychooncology: Psychological Care of the Patient With Cancer. Edited by Holland J, Rowland J. New York, Oxford University Press, 1989, pp 444–454

Massie M, Holland J, Glass E: Delirium in terminally ill cancer patients. Am J Psychiatry 140:148–150, 1983

Massie M, Holland J, Straker N: Psychotherapeutic interventions, in Handbook of Psychooncology: Psychological Care of the Patient With Cancer. Edited by Holland J, Rowland J. New York, Oxford University Press, 1989, pp 273–283

McCrae R: Age differences in the use of coping mechanisms. J Gerontol 37:454–460, 1982

Meadows A, Hobbie W: The medical consequences of cure. Cancer 58:524–528, 1986

Meyers B, Mei-tal V: Psychiatric reactions during tricyclic treatment of the elderly reconsidered. J Clin Psychopharmacol 3:2–6, 1983

Miller P, Richardson J, Jyu C, et al: Association of low serum anticholinergic levels and cognitive impairment in elderly presurgical patients. Am J Psychiatry 145:342–345, 1988

167

Moran M, Thompson T, Nies A: Sleep disorders in the elderly. Am J Psychiatry 145:1369–1378, 1988

Myers W: Dynamic Therapy of the Older Patient. New York, Jason Aronson, 1984

Nemiroff R, Colarusso C: The Race Against Time: Psychotherapy and Psychoanalysis in the Second Half of Life. New York, Plenum, 1985

Nerenz D, Love R, Leventhal H, et al: Psychosocial consequences of cancer chemotherapy for elderly patients. Health Serv Res 20:961–976, 1986

Pasnau R, Fawzy F, Fawzy N: Role of the physician in bereavement. Psychiatr Clin North Am 10:109–120, 1987

Patchell R, Posner J: Neurological complications of systemic cancer. Neurol Clin 3:729–750, 1985

Patterson R, Moon J: Aging, in Handbook of Clinical Behavior Therapy With Adults. Edited by Hensen M, Bellack A. New York, Plenum, 1985, pp 573–601

Pattison E: The experience of dying. Am J Psychother 21:32–43, 1967

Pitts W, Fann W, Sajadi C, et al: Alprazolam in older depressed inpatients. J Clin Psychiatry 44:213–215, 1983

Pollack B, Perel J: Tricyclic antidepressants: contemporary issues for therapeutic practice. Can J Psychiatry 34:609–617, 1989

Rait D, Lederberg M: The family of the cancer patient, in Handbook of Psychooncology: Psychological Care of the Patient With Cancer. Edited by Holland J, Rowland J. New York, Oxford University Press, 1989, pp 585–598

Rapp S, Vrana S: Substituting nonsomatic for somatic symptoms in the diagnosis of depression in elderly male medical patients. Am J Psychiatry 146:1197–1200, 1989

Rennecker R: Countertransference reactions to cancer. Psychosom Med 19:409–418, 1957

Reynolds C, Hoch C, Kupfer D, et al: Bedside differentiation of depressive pseudodementia from dementia. Am J Psychiatry 145:1099–1103, 1988

Rickels K, Feighner J, Smith W: Alprazolam, amitriptyline, doxepin, and placebo in the treatment of depression. Arch Gen Psychiatry 42:703–707, 1985

Roose SP, Glassman AH: Cardiovascular Effects of Tricyclic Antidepressants in Depressed Patients. Journal of Clinical Psychiatry Monograph Series No 7. 1989

Rovner B, David A, Lucas-Blaustein M, et al: Self-care capacity and anticholinergic drug levels in nursing home patients. Am J Psychiatry 145:107–109, 1988

Salzman C: Treatment of the elderly agitated patient. J Clin Psychiatry 48 (suppl):19–22, 1987

Samiy A: Clinical manifestations of disease in the elderly. Med Clin North Am 67:333–344, 1983

Satel S, Nelson J: Stimulants in the treatment of depression: a critical review. J Clin Psychiatry 50:241–249, 1989

Saunders J, Valente S: Cancer and suicide. Oncology Nursing Forum 15:575–581, 1988

Schmale A: Psychological reactions to recurrences or metastases or disseminated cancer. Int J Radiat Oncol Biol Phys 1:515–520, 1976

Schmale A, Morrow G, Schmitt M, et al: Well-being of cancer survivors. Psychosom Med 45:163–169, 1983

Shanfield S: On surviving cancer: psychological considerations. Compr Psychiatry 21:128–134, 1980

Silberfarb P, Greer S: Psychological concomitants of cancer. Am J Psychother 36:470–478, 1982

Silberfarb P, Oxman T: The effects of cancer therapies on the central nervous system. Adv Psychosom Med 18:13–25, 1988

Small G: Tricyclic antidepressants for medically ill geriatric patients. J Clin Psychiatry 50 (suppl):27–33, 1989

Snider E: Awareness and use of health services by the elderly: a Canadian study. Med Care 28:1177–1182, 1980

Spikes J, Holland J: The physicians' response to the dying patient, in Psychological Care of the Medically Ill. Edited by Strain J, Grossman S. Norwalk, CT, Appleton-Century-Crofts, 1975, pp 138–148

Stoudemire A, Riether A: Evaluation and treatment of paranoid syndromes in the elderly: a review. Gen Hosp Psychiatry 9:267–274, 1987

Sussman N: Diagnosis and treatment of anxiety in the elderly. Geriatric Medicine Today 10:1–8, 1988

Tasman A: Loss of self-cohesion in terminal illness. J Am Acad Psychoanal 10:515–526, 1982

Thompson E, Fairclough D, Crom, et al: Normal physical and psychosocial function in the majority of childhood cancer patients surviving 10 years or more from diagnosis. Proceedings of the American Society of Clinical Oncology 6:258, 1987

Tross S, Holland J: Psychological sequelae in cancer survivors, in Handbook of Psychooncology: Psychological Care of the Patient With Cancer. Edited by Holland J, Rowland J. New York, Oxford University Press, 1989, pp 101–116

Vachon M: Unresolved grief in persons with cancer referred for psychotherapy. Psychiatr Clin North Am 10:467–486, 1987

Viederman M: The psychodynamic life narrative: a psychotherapeutic intervention useful in crisis situations. Psychiatry 46:236–246, 1983

Weissman A, Worden J: The existential plight in cancer: significance of the first 100 days. Int J Psychiatry Med 7:1–15, 1976–1977

Welch-McCaffrey D, Hoffman B, Leigh S, et al: Surviving adult cancers, 2: psychosocial implications. Ann Intern Med 111:517–524, 1989

Wilson C, Rimer B, Bennett D, et al: Educating the older cancer patient: obstacles and opportunities. Health Educ Q 10 (suppl):76–87, 1984

Wood K, Harris M, Morreale M, et al: Drug induced psychosis and depression in the elderly. Psychiatr Clin North Am 11:167–193, 1988

Chapter Ten

HYPNOTHERAPY AND OLDER ADULTS

Jonathan Holt, M.D.

In this chapter, I describe the use of hypnotherapy in the treatment of elderly patients. Toward this end, I will first review the phenomenon of hypnosis technique and utilization and follow this with a few clinical examples.

Hypnosis can be best described as an altered state of consciousness with the important characteristic of hypersuggestibility (Hull 1933). J. Braid was the first to demonstrate that hypnosis is a state that occurs in the individual, not a forced interaction between hypnotist and subject (Braid 1852; Kravis 1988). Thus, all hypnosis can be considered a self-hypnotic process that can, on occasion, be guided externally.

The process of facilitation is called a hypnotic induction. There are many different forms of induction, but most include a fixation or manipulation of attention (Brown and Fromm 1986; Hilgard 1977; Wall 1984). Hypnosis shares this characteristic with both meditation techniques and situations of restricted environmental stimulation therapy (REST). To be more specific, a mantra meditation technique such as transcendental meditation (TM) involves attending to a word or syllable, such as "om," and repeating it to oneself again and again. This shift of attention away from ordinary topics of attention by use of the mantra repetition produces the alteration of consciousness characteristic of meditation (Davidson and Goleman 1977). REST manipulates attention by actually physically reducing the sensory input (by using, for example, flotation tanks, sensory isolation chambers, etc.), depriving one of the ordinary objects of attention (Barabasz and Barabasz 1989).

Standard hypnotic inductions are similarly structured (Wall 1984). In the classical inductions, people were instructed to fix their gaze on a crystal or the hypnotist's eyes and to focus their attention on the hypnotist's voice. Hypnosis differs from meditation and REST techniques, however, in the subsequent deepening and utilization phases. The various deepening techniques of hypnosis have in common the offering of complex tasks and imagery that involve the subjects in manipulating and immersing themselves in a new frame of reference or a new "reality orientation" (Shor 1959). For example, a hypnotic subject might be told that he or she is walking down a long, winding staircase that leads to a beach with cool sea breezes. In complying with the above suggestion, the subject would be both building the imagined alternate reality and immersing him- or herself in it. The subject's experience would differ from both waking consciousness and the various levels and experience of consciousness characteristic of one of the classical meditative states (Shor 1959; Tart 1979). There is some indication that the individual's physiological responses in the hypnotic state are also different (Walrath and Hamilton 1975).

CLINICAL ISSUES AND CASE HISTORIES

The uses of hypnosis and hypnotherapy with the older adult do not significantly differ from those with other age groups. Some research has established the fact that hypnotizability scores show stability over long periods of time (see Piccione et al. 1989). One Swedish nursing home study suggests that hypnotizability declines in later adulthood (Berg and Melin 1975). On the other hand, some anecdotal material has shown a slight increase in the capacity of older adults to be hypnotized (T. Hackett, 1983, personal communication). Organicity may be more common and the need for integration and acceptance of life events may loom larger in the older adult. However, in my experience there are no specific issues that are truly limited to this population. There may be some increased need to hand-tailor approaches; for example, one might call on a greater awareness of adult development and life cycle themes. But in all candor, I have not personally found hypnosis with older adults to be qualitatively different. There are no absolute a priori contraindications. Organicity can make hypnosis more difficult, particularly if attention is impaired. Psychosis can make hypnosis more difficult and create complications, but it is not an absolute contraindication. Both extreme mania and depression make hypnosis extremely difficult. Mildly depressed and euthymic or almost euthymic bipolar patients, on the other hand, are workable.

Case 1

The patient was a widow in her late 60s, with fairly severe Parkinson's disease, diabetes, and problems in ambulation. She was beginning to recover from a major depression and had been referred by her neurologist, who felt that she should have been more mobile and generally functional than she was, given the limited extent of her Parkinson's disease. During the previous winter, she had been hospitalized both for Parkinson's disease and for complications of her diabetes. Her doctors had also attempted to treat her depression, but she had a severe delirium in response to a trial of tricyclic antidepressants. The referral was specifically for hypnotherapy and whatever other treatment was required.

When she appeared in my office for the first time, in a wheelchair pushed by one of her sons, she looked older than her stated age and required considerable assistance in transferring to the lounge chair. She clearly had all the stigmata of parkinsonism and, on clinical assessment, was still mildly depressed. After obtaining an initial history from her, I gave a simple explanation of the hypnotic process. In this talk, I emphasized that the process is generally one of self-hypnosis, aided occasionally by external guidance. I did a preliminary induction to illustrate the process to her and then began to teach her self-hypnosis. She was moderately hypnotizable in terms of easily achieved depth of trance. I used a formal, somewhat standardized induction, but I timed my suggestions and tailored my vocal rhythms to coincide with those of the patient in terms of her rate of breathing, muscle tension, body position, and such. I gave her an outline to follow in home practice.

The content of the work varied, but I generally encouraged her to have hypnotic dreams of vivid fantasies in which she saw herself as younger, fully mobile, and full of vigor and enjoyment of life. I used some open-ended projective techniques to assess whether there were special issues regarding family relations, mourning issues, or secondary gain for remaining dysfunctional. These were of little importance, but she did exhibit considerable anxiety about falling and a fear of failure. Specific, realistic rehearsal imagery was used, supplemented with more fantastic imagery of her dancing and flying. Imagery was also used to depict her brain being imbued with renewed vigor. Direct suggestions were alternated with metaphors and indirect suggestion. Suggestions were also given that her unconscious would know what to do and would temper her attempts at action with whatever modicum of prudence was required.

This therapy continued over the course of several months. Sessions were dependent on her children's schedules, so that the scheduling was somewhat erratic. The patient's depressive symptoms abated entirely. Her locomotion improved until she was able to ambulate alone and unaided. At this point, the patient chose to terminate treatment.

173

This case has a sequel. Some time after termination, the patient fell and broke her hip. Her family called me in to consult with her while she was still in the hospital following a hip pinning. They were concerned that her depression might recur.

When I first saw her in the hospital, she was in considerable discomfort. I worked with her in a trance state to decrease the discomfort, using both direct and indirect suggestions. Initially, the patient achieved an impressive (though not complete) analgesia. Her pain suddenly returned a few days later, however, during physical therapy. Radiological examination revealed that there was a complication from the first procedure: a second fracture around the pin. She was returned to surgery for a second, more radical procedure. Several months of traction in the hospital ensued.

When the patient started to have a serious recurrence of her major depression, I decided to treat it with nortriptyline, beginning with very small doses in the hope of avoiding side effects. She quickly developed a delirium, however, which subsided on cessation of the tricyclic treatment. Rather than attempting to treat her with a combination of medications, I resorted to hypnotherapy again. I used both indirect and direct suggestions to promulgate healing and to aid in normalization of her mood. Despite a long hospitalization, the patient recovered from her depression and maintained her level of confidence. She was discharged from the hospital and was able to walk again with the aid of a walker. I might add here that this time I placed special emphasis on suggestions and imagery that stressed prudent efforts to rein in some of her impatient attempts to do more than was feasible.

The analgesia work is illustrative of hypnoanalgesic phenomena. If there is some physical need for pain, the hypnotically attained analgesia may be incomplete or may stop (in this case, when the new fracture appeared) (Hilgard 1975). I have seen this phenomenon a number of times in my practice. In one instance involving a woman in labor, the analgesia suddenly stopped. It was subsequently discovered that at that moment she had developed an abruption. This illustrates the self-protective processes at work in hypnosis.

Case 2

The second patient was a single woman in her late 70s, who suffered from a major depression and had made a serious suicide attempt by ingesting an overdose of antidepressants and other medications. Her friends had found her in a comatose state several days after the attempt, and she was hospitalized in an intensive care unit for over a week. A decubitus ulcer incurred during the period of coma had led to severe necrotic damage in one leg. After coming out of the coma, the patient was transferred to the psychiatric hospital for treatment of the depression and for surgical follow-up for the decubitus ulcer. I supplemented her psychopharmacological treatments with hypnotherapy. I might add here that in this patient's background, there was a dismaying history of depression and successful suicide (one parent, two grandparents, several siblings, and some cousins).

On initial assessment, the patient was only mildly to moderately hypnotizable. She was rationalistic and analytical, a clear example of what the Spiegels called "Apollonian" (Spiegel and Spiegel 1978). I spent a particularly long period of time with her explaining hypnotic phenomena. I found it useful to describe some of the work on cerebral laterality and the importance of the "nonlinear," "holistic" right hemisphere. This gave the patient a rationale (or permission) for allowing herself to experience nonrational thought processes.

I used a structured induction. However, in the initial phase, I spent more time and put in some extra deepening exercises. I also did a number of inductions within a session to give the patient practice and to get feedback from her about what she experienced as most effective. While many people find it easier to use more fantastic imagery (Shone 1982), this woman felt more comfortable in using true-to-life visualizations. The main treatment modality I used with her was semistructured, guided imagery. This allowed her ample opportunity to visualize her body and mind healing in different ways. I directed her unconscious mind to seek out multiple ways in which to find meaning in her life, and I suggested that she develop a powerful sense of purpose in the aspects of her life in which her physical activity might become limited. I emphasized future pacing techniques whereby the patient imagined that she was in a future time and was telling someone how she had managed to achieve such a miraculous recovery. I instructed her to have nocturnal dreams on the subject to find new solutions to her difficulties that she would later use. I also utilized open-ended visualizations to scan for underlying concerns that she might be too "polite" and controlled to mention spontaneously. I felt that this technique would be of particular importance, given the fact that she had attempted suicide while under the care of an outpatient psychiatrist and without having given him warning.

Using these methods, the patient made a rapid recovery from her depressive symptoms and gained considerable insight into existential and adult development issues. Her decubitus ulcer also healed. Follow-up over the ensuing year and a half has shown good maintenance of the progress made.

This case illustrates the usefulness of hand-tailoring hypnotic techniques and suggestions. It also illustrates the use of hypnosis and hypnotherapy as an adjunct to psychopharmacological treatment.

Case 3

The patient was a widower in his mid-70s who was referred by his children for therapy. He had suffered a cerebrovascular accident with resultant motor difficulties. As in the first case described above, the patient's doctors felt that the man's ambulation could be improved. His family reported that he had been anxious much of his life and had suffered from multiple phobias and obsessions. His anxieties after his stroke centered on ambulation. Specifically, he worried that he might fall or would be unable to cope with particular physical challenges, such as using the bathroom. He was reported to have suffered some cognitive impairment, both after the stroke and subsequent to various medication trials. His family had urged his physician to take him off all but the most essential medications, and the physician had reluctantly complied.

On the first visit, the patient came escorted and physically supported by his chauffeur. He was pleasant but extremely anxious, and he did not meet criteria for depression, either overt or masked. From his history, I learned that his anxiety had occasionally reached panic proportions. On assessment, he was only mildly hypnotizable. I suggested that he might benefit from tricyclic antidepressant treatment for his anxiety and panic symptoms, but he wished to discuss this with his personal physician and his family first. However, he did agree to undergo hypnotherapy for his anxieties and to help improve his physical performance.

It was quite difficult to induce a trance, either by enhanced standard inductions or by Ericksonian methods (Erickson 1980). He would compulsively fidget or would suddenly open his eyes and begin to talk about one subject or another, clearly emerging from the trance. In response to this, I decided to try a combined approach with three main components: careful initial explanations of what the process would involve; an authoritarian stance, with strict instructions not to move, fidget, or open his eyes once they were closed until I explicitly gave him permission to do so; and Ericksonian pacing of his breathing and other rhythms and surveying of his muscle tone for an assessment of the level of his trance. I also used a mixture of projective techniques, general guided imagery to promote his confidence and improve his motor and ambulatory performance, and more specific behavior modification methods geared to desensitize him concerning his anxieties about falling and being able to cope physically. I instructed him in self-hypnosis, gave him a crib sheet, and told him to keep records of his attempts at self-hypnosis. I later supplemented this with in vivo practice sessions involving ambulation in my office, in the corridors, and on the grounds of the hospital. At a later date, when he had made considerable progress, his family consented to his taking low-dose tricyclic antidepressants. His improvement continued, and by the time we terminated, he was regularly walking by himself (albeit, at times, with the use of a quad cane), attending various social and family functions, and even beginning to date. His family reported that his mentation had also considerably improved.

The usefulness of tailoring induction methods to the patient is again illustrated here. One of the interesting aspects of this case is that the patient was able to work in treatment to improve, despite the presence of moderate cognitive deficits. It also demonstrates the utility of combining different therapeutic techniques, including trance work and real-life practice methods. In this case, I did assessments in both the waking and trance states for the presence of feelings of bereavement, which I feel is important not to overlook in patients in this age group.

Case 4

In a somewhat parallel case, I was asked by a widow to treat her feelings of panic when driving an automobile. These feelings had started about 3 months after the sudden death of her husband from a heart attack some 5 years earlier. My initial plan was to treat her with a combination of in-trance desensitization and in vivo practice work. She denied any unresolved feelings of grief. Initial trance work went well but somewhat slowly. I used an open-ended fishing technique: "Imagine yourself in a pleasant meadow with a pool of water. Look into the pool and see what reflections are there." She spontaneously saw an image of her husband. This evolved into in-trance work, in which she had conversations with him and his image gave her a blessing. Though she did not spontaneously improve, the other work began to accelerate at that point and she was able to leave treatment free of symptoms.

What developed in this case as a spontaneous phenomenon has been developed by others as a formal technique. Jung (1961) used the technique of having conversations with imaginary figures or archetypes. Cerney (1989) has created therapy programs at the Menninger Clinic, where patients are encouraged to have in-trance conversations and guided interactions with deceased significant others.

Case 5

The patient was a widow in her 70s, who had had a recent stroke and a 30-plus-year history of bipolar illness. She had been maintained on lithium until her stroke, when the drug was discontinued. She had also been treated with tricyclic antidepressants, but these, too, had been stopped because of arrhythmias. She subsequently had a series of psychiatric hospitalizations, which led to her being put back on both lithium and a tricyclic antidepressant. Her management was complicated by the fact that she insisted on being discharged to her home, where she was unable to cope adequately. When she again decompensated and was hospitalized at our hospital, she was treated pharmacologically. When she restabilized, two things happened: 1) we arranged for her to be discharged to a nursing home, and 2) I taught her self-hypnosis and did a number of exercises with her.

Once she became sufficiently adept at self-hypnosis, I suggested that she review her recent past in altered hypnotic time. I then suggested that her mind would offer her a metaphor or symbol of harmony and balance in her life. Interestingly, she described a scene in which she was sitting on a child's swing but was balanced and still. I further suggested to her that her unconscious could take that metaphor, build on it, and use it. Shortly after this, she was discharged from the hospital. While the nursing home placement was, in all likelihood, the key intervention, the hypnotic suggestions must have also been instrumental in keeping the patient out of a psychiatric hospital for the past 3 years. Previously, she had been averaging several hospitalizations a year.

Bipolar illness is a particular challenge for hypnotherapy. In general, most experts do not recommend using this technique (Brown and Fromm 1986). However, this and other cases I have seen indicate that hypnotherapy may have a role with the euthymic bipolar patient in helping to maintain stability in that state.

While this last case involves only a minor use of hypnosis, it illustrates some of the benefits of the hypnotic context in treatments primarily devoted to other modalities.

Case 6

The patient was a man in his mid-70s with a history of late onset, recurrent psychotic depressions. He had responded once to electroconvulsive therapy (ECT) and then had been discharged on tricyclic antidepressants. His home life was unstable, however, because of his shrewish and character-disordered wife. He did not remain compliant with his treatment regimen and suffered a relapse. This led both to his being rehospitalized and retreated with ECT and to a remission of symptoms. On this occasion, family work involved the patient and his children. He was able to give his wife an ultimatum to the effect that either she get into treatment or he would not return home. She refused to comply, and the patient went to stay with one of his children. He did quite well on medication, supportive therapy, and family sessions with his children. However, he was conflicted about remaining apart from his wife, who was becoming increasingly dysfunctional.

The key modalities of his outpatient treatment had always been pharmacotherapy paired with supportive and occasional insight-oriented therapy. The patient's largest gains had always come from either biological treatment or family sessions and strategic interventions. He had a penchant for answering questions with questions. At one point, when he was again agonizing over whether to return to his wife, I stopped his talk and told him to shut his eyes. Without calling it hypnosis, I told him to relax, take some slow deep breaths, and then to imagine himself where he wanted to be in 6 months. At first, he reopened his eyes and said: "Well you know, I'm not sure. I'd like——." I then interrupted him and repeated my instructions. After a pause, he said, "I see myself at my son's house and I'm happy." From that point on, there was essentially no further vacillation, and the patient has continued to do well in the ensuing 2 years.

It is not clear whether one can consider this to be hypnosis. Though little effort was put into the induction, the context was similar to that seen in hypnosis. The patient was no longer looking at me or his son (who was present) and was no longer talking about other things. Rather, he had switched over into a mode in which he was imagining and experiencing things directly and was more open to spontaneous imagery and intuition. Even if one chooses not to use hypnotic techniques specifically, it may be useful to borrow something occasionally from the hypnotic context, especially the switch from talking about something to imagining and experiencing it vividly.

CONCLUDING REMARKS

In this chapter, I have offered an introduction to the phenomenon of hypnosis and a taste for its potential as an adjunct to various therapies with the older adult. Again, it is important to emphasize that the utilizations are essentially the same as those in other age groups. It is not within the purview of this chapter to prepare the reader to go out and practice these techniques. Rather, I recommend that, if interested, the reader pursue larger works on the subject or even undergo training.

REFERENCES

Barabasz A, Barabasz M: Effects of restricted environmental stimulation: enhancement of hypnotizability for experimental and chronic pain control. Int J Clin Exp Hypn 27(3):217–231, 1989

Berg S, Melin E: Hypnotic susceptibility in old age: some data from residential homes for old people. Int J Clin Exp Hypn 23(30):184–189, 1975

Braid J: Magic, Witchcraft, Animal Magnetism, Hypnotism, and Electrobiology: Being a Digest of the Latest Views of the Author on These Subjects. London, John Churchill, 1852

Brown D, Fromm E: Hypnotherapy and Hypnoanalysis. Hillsdale, NJ, Lawrence Erlbaum Associates, 1986

Cerney M: Paper presented to the 40th annual scientific meeting of the Society for Clinical and Experimental Hypnosis, St. Louis, MO, November 1989

Davidson RJ, Goleman D: The role of attention in meditation and hypnosis: a psychobiological perspective on transformations of consciousness. Int J Clin Exp Hypn 25(4):291–308, 1977

Erickson M: The Collected Papers of M.H. Erickson (4 vols). Edited by Rossi E. New York, Irvington Press, 1980

Hilgard E: Divided Consciousness. New York, John Wiley, 1977, 1989

Hilgard E, Hilgard J: Hypnosis in the Relief of Pain. Los Altos, CA, William Kaufman, 1975

Hull C: Hypnosis and Suggestibility. New York, Irvington, 1933

Jung C: Memories, Dreams, and Reflections. New York, Random House, 1961

Kravis N: James Braid's psychophysiology: a turning point in the history of dynamic psychiatry. Am J Psychiatry 145:1191–1206, 1988

Piccione C, Hilgard E, Zimbardo P: On the degree of stability of measured hypnotizability over a 25-year period. J Pers Soc Psychol 56:289–295, 1989

Shone R: Autohypnosis. Northhamptonshire, England, Thorsons, 1982

Shor R: Hypnosis and the concept of the generalized reality orientation. Am J Psychother 13:582–602, 1959

Spiegel H, Spiegel D: Trance and Treatment: Clinical Uses of Hypnosis. New York, Basic Books, 1978

Tart C: States of Consciousness. New York, EP Dutton, 1979

Wall T: Hypnotic phenomena, in Clinical Hypnosis. Edited by Wester W, Smith A. Philadelphia, PA, JB Lippincott, 1984

Walrath L, Hamilton D: Autonomic correlates of meditation and hypnosis. Am J Clin Hypn 17(3):190–197, 1975

IMPACT OF A BEHAVIOR THERAPY ON THE PSYCHOLOGICAL STATUS OF INCONTINENT ELDERLY NURSING HOME RESIDENTS: QUANTITATIVE AND QUALITATIVE ASSESSMENT

Lucy C. Yu, Ph.D., D. Lynne Kaltreider, M.Ed., Teh-wei Hu, Ph.D., and W. Edward Craighead, Ph.D.

The aging of the American population is one of the most compelling future demographic trends facing health care providers. Increasing longevity has made the population 75 years of age and older more numerous in both absolute and relative terms. The unprecedented increased size of the elderly population ages 65 and older in the United States, especially during recent years, has resulted mainly from decreased mortality among the elderly.

One consequence of this decreased mortality is increased morbidity among those aged 75 and older. Advanced age and multiple chronic conditions eventually force many elderly people to be institutionalized. One of the major problems of people in institutions is urinary incontinence. Urinary incontinence is costly in personal, psychological, physical, and financial terms.

Urinary incontinence is one of the most prevalent clinical conditions experienced by elderly people. About 9% of the elderly in the community experience some urinary incontinence (Harris 1986), as

---

This study was supported by the National Institute on Aging and the National Center for Nursing Research. We thank Dr. Jessie F. Igou for training the nursing research assistants, and Drs. Thomas J. Rohner and Patrick J. Dennis for the urological evaluations.

do 40–50% of the elderly in nursing homes (Hu et al. 1984; Ouslander et al. 1987; Yarnell and St. Leger 1979). It is estimated that in the United States about 800,000 elderly in nursing homes and 2.5 million elderly in the community are incontinent (Hu 1986). Several studies suggest that, in addition to the psychological stress it causes, incontinence alone costs nursing homes from $2–4 billion annually, which represents at least 10% of total nursing home care costs (Brazda 1983; Hu 1986, 1989; Ouslander and Kane 1983).

Although urinary incontinence is often viewed as a biological disease entity, it can result from multiple etiological mechanisms (Brocklehurst et al. 1968; Diokno 1986; Freeman and Baxby 1982; Resnick and Yalla 1985; Willington 1975). Health professionals and patients alike often mistakenly view the condition as a necessary part of aging (Mitteness 1983). Nevertheless, the stigma attached to urinary incontinence can have serious consequences for the psychological well-being and social functioning of adults (Ory et al. 1986; Yu and Kaltreider 1987). Wilson (1948) suggested that incontinence implies an indignity to the social integrity of the individual. Willington (1975) found that incontinent elderly displayed evidence of psychological trauma characterized by declining control and increasing dependence. The social and personal isolation that results from incontinence, in combination with feelings of guilt, fear, shame, and helplessness, may even lead to clinical depression (Spiro 1978; Wells 1984; Willington 1975; Yu 1986).

In this chapter, we will assess psychological change associated with the treatment effects of a behavior therapy for urinary incontinence. Specifically, we will explore how a behavior therapy program affected the psychological well-being of incontinent women in nursing homes. We hypothesized that behavior therapy would improve both the incontinence status and the psychological and affective status of patients.

Older persons characteristically suffer from multiple, complex medical problems and chronic conditions. Our past technological achievements have done little to improve the day-to-day experience of most elders in long-term care institutions, where nursing care rather than the application of recently developed therapeutic interventions dominates residents' lives. Using a behavior therapy program to help elderly residents reduce urinary incontinence is a noninvasive technique that may be integrated with nursing care to ameliorate this condition. This chapter reports on the psychological effects of combining a behavior therapy program with nursing care to reduce the frequency of urinary incontinence.

METHOD

Population and Sample

One hundred thirty-three incontinent elderly women from seven central Pennsylvania nursing homes participated in a randomized clinical trial to evaluate the effectiveness of a behavior therapy (prompted toileting) program on participants' urinary incontinence and psychological status.

After giving informed consent, 143 women first qualified for the prompted toileting program and were assigned randomly to treatment and control groups. To qualify for participation, residents had to be incontinent on average at least once every other day (0.5 wet episodes per day) during 3 weeks of baseline observation, undergo a urodynamic evaluation by the project urologists, be female, be aged 65 or older, and be able to give informed consent. Ten of the 143 subjects did not complete the 13-week behavior therapy period because they died, voluntarily withdrew, or were transferred, hospitalized, or catheterized. We were able to obtain pre- and postscores for 84% of the participants on the Mini-Mental State Exam (MMSE) (Folstein et al. 1975), for 83% on the Center for Epidemiological Studies Depression Scale (CES-D) (Radloff 1977), and for 81% on the Psychological General Well-Being Scale (PGWB) (Duprey 1978). The outcome of these measures forms the basis of this chapter.

Table 11-1 presents the sociodemographic characteristics of the sample ($n = 133$) during the 3-week baseline period. The average age of the participants was 85.4 years, 98% were white, and 82% were widowed. About one-third had less than a high school education, about one-fourth graduated from high school, less than one-tenth had some college education, and one-fourth did not answer questions about their education. Fifty-three percent of the participants were incontinent when admitted to the nursing home: 25% were admitted to the nursing home with urinary incontinence; 27% had dual incontinence. Forty percent of the participants had been in the home for 1 to 3 years; however, the average length of stay of the participants was 4 years.

Table 11-2 shows the functional status and medical diagnoses of the overall sample. Most of the participants were reported to need assistance with their activities of daily living—bathing, dressing, transferring, eating, and using the toilet. Only 8% were reported able to toilet without assistance.

The women in the study had a number of chronic conditions, the

Table 11-1. Sociodemographic characteristics of individuals recruited and retained in the study (all women)

Characteristic	Experimental group ($n = 65$) (%)	Control group ($n = 68$) (%)	Total sample ($n = 133$) (%)
Age			
< 65	3	0	1
65–69	0	4	2
70–74	5	6	5
75–79	6	12	8
80–84	25	19	22
85–89	31	24	28
90–94	25	24	24
95 and older	6	12	9
Mean age (years)	85.6	85.3	85.4
Standard error of mean	0.861	0.942	0.602
Ethnic background			
Black	2	1	1
White	98	96	97
Other	0	1	1
Marital status			
Married	8	10	8
Widowed	82	76	80
Divorced	5	6	6
Never married	5	6	5
Education			
Less than high school	33	31	31
High school graduate	29	18	24
College	12	10	12
Don't know	22	31	25
Incontinence status upon admission			
Urinary incontinent only	22	26	25
Fecal incontinent only	3	7	5
Both urinary and fecal incontinent	26	26	27
Neither urinary nor fecal incontinent	45	38	40
Level of care			
Skilled	22	24	22
Intermediate	77	74	77
Years from date of admission			
< 1	20	19	21
1–3	49	34	40
4–6	12	21	17
7–9	5	15	10
10 or more	9	9	9
Mean years	3.4	4.5	4.0
Standard error of mean	0.457	0.543	0.356

Note. Columns may not add to 100% due to rounding errors and missing responses.

184

Table 11-2. Functional status and medical diagnosis

	Experimental group ($n = 65$) (%)	Control group ($n = 68$) (%)	Total sample ($n = 133$) (%)
Dependency in pre-ADL components			
Bathing	80	90	85
Dressing	86	94	90
Transferring	88	90	89
Feeding	66	76	71
Incontinent (fecal or urinary)	100	100	100
Toileting	89	96	92
Katz ADL dependency score			
Dependent in 1 function	8	0	4
Dependent in 2 functions	3	1	2
Dependent in 3 functions	2	3	2
Dependent in 4 functions	9	7	8
Dependent in 5 functions	17	22	20
Dependent in 6 functions	62	62	62
Mean score[a]	5.1	5.5	5.3
Standard error of mean	0.188	0.110	0.109
Current medical diagnosis[b]			
Cardiorespiratory	83	76	80
Hardening of the arteries	62	58	60
High blood pressure	26	31	29
Gastrointestinal	22	19	20
Constipation	19	15	17
Ulcers	2	6	4
Genitourinary	13	12	12
Kidney trouble/chronic urinary tract infections	12	12	12
Neurological	80	81	80
Stroke/cerebral vascular accident	6	10	8
Other circulatory problems	23	15	19
Organic brain syndrome	25	15	20
Senile dementia	29	31	30
Musculoskeletal	60	46	53
Arthritis/rheumatism	49	39	44

Note: Columns may not add to 100% due to rounding errors and missing responses. The data in this table were provided by the nursing home.
[a]0 = total independence, 6 = total dependence.
[b]Most patients had multiple diagnoses: the range was 2 to 11; the mean number of diagnoses was 4.

185

most often cited being arteriosclerosis (60%), hypertension (29%), senile dementia (30%), and arthritis (44%). Many of the participants had more than one chronic disease or condition and multiple disabilities. The average number of medical diagnoses was 4.3 per patient; the range was from 2 to 11 (Yu et al. 1988).

TREATMENTS

Behavior Therapy Procedure

The behavior therapy used in this study is based on basic psychological principles of behavioral change (Craighead 1981). Two specific principles underlie this particular behavior therapy: the prompting of individuals to toilet at regularly scheduled intervals (in this case, hourly), and social reinforcement for appropriate toileting behavior. A nursing research assistant (NRA) checked each participating resident each hour from 7 A.M. to 9 P.M. to determine her wet/dry status. The NRA then asked and prompted the resident to toilet, assisted the resident to the toilet if necessary, praised the resident for successful toileting, and provided social reinforcement in the form of special attention (i.e., conversation or additional personal services) if the resident was found dry on the scheduled check. If the resident asked to go to the toilet before the prompt was administered at the hourly check, the prompt was not given but the resident was toileted and appropriately reinforced. Subjects were encouraged to hold their urine until the next hourly check but were told that if they needed to use the toilet other than at the scheduled toileting time, they should call the NRA so that appropriate assistance could be provided and data recorded.

The social reinforcement (time and conversation) given for staying dry was designed to produce the behavioral change associated with adaptive and appropriate voiding patterns. There has been extensive research demonstrating the use and effectiveness of behavioral procedures for enuresis with children (Parker and Whitehead 1982), but employing such techniques with elderly people has only begun recently. Although these reinforcement measures have been used in several training programs for incontinent elderly (Burgio and Burgio 1986; Schnelle 1983), this study was one of the first clinical trials. As the program was consistently implemented, residents developed an increased physical ability to control their voiding, an increased sense of control or self-efficacy (Bandura 1977) over their toileting practices, and an increased motivation to toilet appropriately. The patients' response to this behavior therapy program is described in Kaltreider et al. (1990).

Control Procedure

The women in the control group also were checked hourly by the NRAs to determine their incontinence status. When a control participant was found wet, the NRA notified the regular nursing home aide. Participants in the control group were not prompted to toilet by the NRAs, and they were not given any incontinence-related care by the NRAs. Otherwise, these residents received the usual treatment and nursing care of the regular nursing home staff.

REDUCTION OF INCONTINENCE

Our data indicate that the behavior therapy program was effective in reducing the incidence of incontinence among the women in the treatment group. The program produced a significant reduction in urinary incontinence when it was compared with the "treatment as usual" control group (see Figure 11-1). Seventy-two percent of the treatment women reduced their wet episodes, on average, by 26 percent below their baseline level. (See Hu et al. 1989 for a detailed analysis of the outcome of this study.) The findings indicate that trainees with a high frequency of incontinence improved more than individuals with less severe incontinence. Individuals who were functioning at a higher cognitive level, as measured by their MMSE scores, improved more than those with low levels of cognitive functioning. Individuals with normal bladder capacity responded better to the program than other types of individuals. Totally dependent individuals—those who needed assistance with their activities of daily living—benefited more from the program than less dependent individuals. These identified individual characteristics should be helpful in future implementation of behavior therapy for urinary incontinence.

PSYCHOLOGICAL ASSESSMENT

It was hypothesized that in addition to reducing incontinence, the behavior therapy program would affect the participants' mental and psychological status. Specifically, it was hypothesized that, compared with the control group, 1) the treatment group would have better psychological general well-being after treatment and 2) the

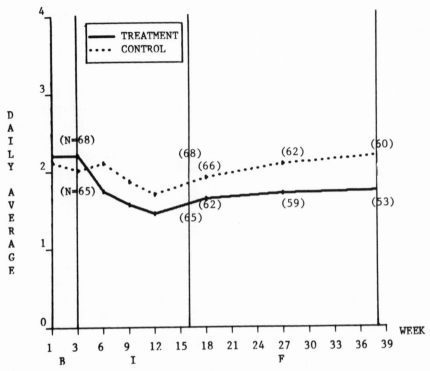

Figure 11-1. Average number of wet episodes per 14-hour day (7 A.M.–9 P.M.) in the treatment (*solid line*) and control (*dotted line*) groups. Reprinted with permission from Hu TW, Igou JF, Kaltreider DL, et al: A clinical trial of a behavioral therapy to reduce urinary incontinence in nursing homes: outcome and implications. JAMA 261:2656–2662, 1989. Copyright 1989, American Medical Association.

treatment group would register fewer depressive symptoms after treatment.

This project was part of a larger collaborative clinical trial studying the effects of various treatments for incontinence. The study used three measures of cognitive and psychological functioning and general well-being: the MMSE (Folstein et al. 1975), the CES-D (Radloff 1977), and the PGWB (Duprey 1978). The National Institute on Aging, the National Center for Nursing Research, and the project's monitoring board recommended use of the MMSE and the CES-D to assess cognitive functioning and depression, and the project added the PGWB to measure the participants' psychological status.

Procedure

The instruments were administered by specially trained research project assistants during the baseline period (pre) and during the 11th week (post) of the 13-week treatment program. These assistants read the items on each instrument to the patients, who had a large-print version of each instrument in front of them. The posttest was administered 2 weeks before the completion of treatment because of concern that patients might become temporarily upset (depressed) at the time the treatment program stopped. Post hoc assessments of patients' status were completed by the NRAs following treatment to provide *qualitative* data for assessing psychological outcomes.

The MMSE is a 30-item interview used to measure cognitive functioning. It may be administered by clinical or lay personnel with little training and usually takes less than 5 minutes to administer. Its brevity and ease of administration make the MMSE a suitable instrument for ascertaining disturbances of cognitive functions. The MMSE has a test-retest reliability of .89 and an interrater reliability of .82. It has been used in clinical settings, and studies have shown that it discriminates the cognitively impaired. It can be scored on a scale of 0–30. Folstein et al. (1975) suggest that patients who score 23 or below have severe symptoms of impairment.

The CES-D is a self-report 20-item scale that groups symptoms of depression into negative and positive affect, somatic and retarded activity, and interpersonal items. Subjects are first asked whether they feel depressed; if the answer is no, respondents are assigned a zero score. If the answer is yes, the interviewer then probes for the degree of depression; respondents are assigned a score of 1 to 3, depending on the severity of the depressive symptoms, to check how often they experienced these symptoms during the preceding week. Therefore, the response categories range from 0–3, with the values of the positive response categories being scored in a reverse direction. The total score is the sum across all 20 items, and it ranges from 0–60, with higher scores indicating greater depressive symptomatology. Researchers suggested a cutoff score of 17 or more to designate an individual as depressed (Radloff 1977). The internal consistency of the CES-D for patient sample is .90; its 4-week test-retest reliability is .67. The CES-D has discriminated well between psychiatric inpatients and general population samples, and has discriminated moderately among levels of severity within patient groups.

The PGWB tests patients' psychological well-being over the preceding 3 months. This scale is designed to assess self-representation of subjective well-being and distress. It measures both affective and cognitive processes. Developed by Duprey (1978) for the National Center for Health Statistics, it was used as part of a national health examination of 6,931 adults aged 24–74 years in 1975. The internal consistency coefficient for the schedule was .93 ($n = 6,931$). Test-retest with up to 3 months separation shows a reliability coefficient of .80. Two field tests have validated this scale as an appropriate instrument to discriminate mental health patients from a community sample at large (Duprey, June 1988, personal communication).

QUANTITATIVE RESULTS AND DISCUSSION

The psychological and mental status data collected during the baseline period and during the 11th week of behavior therapy implementation are shown on Table 11-3. A large portion of the treatment group—42%—was severely cognitively impaired at pretest (scored ≤ 10 on the MMSE), another 23% scored between 11 and 17, and 17% showed moderate cognitive impairment. Only 18% scored 24 or higher—the score that, according to Folstein et al. (1975), signifies no cognitive impairment.

Before treatment, 54% of the control group had severe cognitive impairment, 19% showed much cognitive impairment, 21% showed moderate cognitive impairment, and only 6% had scores that indicated no cognitive impairment. However, further analysis showed no differences between the treatment and control group.

Because of the significant degree of cognitive impairment in our sample, it seemed important to determine the relationship between MMSE scores and depression as reported on the CES-D. The percentages of depressed individuals were almost identical for those who scored less than 24, less than 17, or less than 10 on the MMSE; these are all categories that signify cognitive impairment. In each case, about 32% of the women in these categories had a CES-D score of ≥ 17, indicating depression (cf. Radloff 1977). Among the women who had no cognitive impairment (women who scored ≥ 24 on the MMSE), a higher percentage—45%—reported being depressed (CES-D ≥ 17).

Perhaps the best explanation for these data is that those women who scored over 24 on the MMSE were more in touch with psychological feeling and affect. Cognitively impaired persons appear less likely to report depressive symptoms; unfortunately, no interview or clinical rating data regarding clinical depression are available for comparison purposes. As noted, MMSE predicted outcome on the incontinence variable. Those whose MMSE score was ≥ 10 improved their continence more than those with MMSE scores < 10 ($P = .001$,

190

Table 11-3. Cognitive and psychological characteristics (pre- and posttest scores)

Test and scale	Treatment group (n = 65)		Control group (n = 68)		Total sample (n = 133)	
	Pre (%)	Post (%)	Pre (%)	Post (%)	Pre (%)	Post (%)
Mini-Mental State Exam (MMSE)	(n = 60)		(n = 52)		(n = 112)	
0–10 (severe cognitive impairment)	42	28	54	42	47	35
11–17 (much cognitive impairment)	23	37	19	29	21	33
18–23 (moderate cognitive impairment)	17	23	21	21	19	22
24+ (no cognitive impairment)	18	12	6	8	13	10
Mean score	13.9	14.5	11.3	12.4	12.7	13.5
Standard error of mean	1.028	0.934	1.092	1.051	0.755	0.703
Center for Epidemiological Studies– Depression (CES-D)	(n = 58)		(n = 52)		(n = 110)	
≥ 17 (depressed)	34	41	46	44	40	43
≤ 16 (not depressed)	66	59	54	56	60	57
Mean score	13.5	17.0	16.3	16.1	14.8	16.6
Standard error of mean	1.118	1.370	1.507	1.462	0.930	0.996
Psychological General Well-Being (PGWB)	(n = 58)		(n = 49)		(n = 107)	
6–60 (severe distress)	34	33	39	35	36	34
61–72 (moderate distress)	29	24	14	18	22	22
73–110 (positive well-being)	36	43	47	47	41	44
Mean score	67.2	67.6	67.2	67.4	67.2	67.5
Standard error of mean	2.437	2.513	2.872	2.755	1.855	1.848

Note. Columns may not add to 100% due to rounding errors and missing responses.

two-tailed test), based on the separate regression results from the two subsamples (Hu et al. 1989).

On the measure of general well-being, over one-third (36%) of the sample showed severe distress on the PGWB, about one-fifth (22%) were moderately distressed, and 41% showed positive well-being. (PGWB scores were available for 85% of the total sample.) The average score for the group was 67.1, indicating moderate distress. Normative data indicate that the mean depression score for the older age group (65–74 years) is 8.4, SD = 7.7 (National Center for Health Statistics 1980). For PGWB scores, 74% of a national sample reported positive well-being, 16% reported problems indicative of stress, and 10% reported clinically significant distress (U.S. Health Resources Administration 1977). It appears that the study sample is more depressed and distressed than the general elderly population.

Three separate 2 (pre-post) by 2 (treatment versus control) analyses of variance with repeated measures for the pre-post factor were conducted for the MMSE, CES-D, and PGWB. The results indicated no significant ($P > .05$) treatment, trial, or interaction effects for the MMSE and PGWB. Although the behavior therapy program significantly reduced urinary incontinence, it had no corollary effects on the psychological well-being variables used in this study. Thus, our hypothesis that behavior therapy would improve the effective status of patients was not supported.

A number of issues make it difficult to interpret the results of the psychological data for our patients who were very old (average age 85.6), cognitively and functionally impaired, and incontinent for a number of years. First, one cannot be sure of the effects of the passage of time (13 weeks) on the cognitive status of the frail elderly.

Second, the CES-D and PGWB were not developed and have not been validated for the old-old age group (Weiss 1986); they may not be appropriate instruments for elderly patients who are as cognitively impaired as those in our study. Other instruments or perhaps other methods (e.g., clinical ratings) of evaluating psychological general well-being and affects may prove more valid and valuable among this age group.

The PGWB questionnaire also proved to be problematic. Its format with questions followed by five possible responses is difficult to administer to the very old. Participants had trouble seeing, hearing, understanding, and remembering what had been asked of them. Such impairments were a potential confound for all of the instruments. Some participants simply refused to answer or got tired of answering.

A third important factor is that incontinence in nursing homes is highly correlated with physical and functional impairment. Nursing home patients may be facing other problems at the same time; that is, urinary incontinence may not be their major problem. Incontinence can be extremely stressful, but when it is one of many conditions that elderly patients have to face (some potentially life threatening), this particular dysfunction may seem minor. If this is true, then an improvement in this one aspect of their lives may not be sufficient to affect these patients' general mental and psychological status.

A final potential difficulty in interpreting these data is that the length of time these women have been incontinent may also moderate their specific distress in response to it. We could not obtain information on how long the project participants had been incontinent, but a cursory survey revealed that many had been incontinent for more than 3 years. During a pilot study, cognitively intact patients with urinary incontinence were pretested on the Incontinence Stress Questionnaire-Patient (ISQ-P), an instrument developed to measure psychological stress associated with urinary incontinence. These patients exhibited extremely stressful behaviors, including crying and depressive symptoms (Yu 1986). The respondents in the current study may have been very distressed when their incontinence first began, but after a period of time, when they have so many other things wrong with them, they may learn to tolerate this condition. This may be true for this older age group; incontinence is particularly distressing for the younger elderly, who face fewer life-threatening diseases. Mitteness and Wood (1983) and Ory and colleagues (1986) suggest that older elderly women may simply view incontinence as part of normal aging and in conjunction with other, more serious illnesses with which they deal (Mitteness 1983).

QUALITATIVE RESULTS AND DISCUSSION

So far, this chapter has shown that, for various reasons, we were unable to document statistically significant changes in the psychosocial status of the participants in the behavior therapy program using the standardized instruments administered. Yet members of the project team observed psychological and social well-being changes on the part of some treatment women.

To try to document these changes, at least impressionistically, at the end of the 13-week implementation period at each participating nursing home, we asked each NRA (project staff) to complete a written assessment for each participant with whom she had worked in the treatment group. This assessment asked the NRA to rate each participant in three areas: functional, cognitive, and incontinence. Although the NRAs were not trained in observation techniques, nor did they have professional backgrounds in psychology, they all had experience as nursing aides in long-term care prior to this project, and for 13 consecutive weeks, they had hourly contact during 7-hour shifts with the treatment women in the study.

This section focuses on the project staff's assessments of the social and psychological functioning of the study participants. The project staff were asked to assess whether the subject improved in alertness, stayed about the same, or regressed. If they selected "improved in alertness," they were asked to rate the subject further on the categories of behavioral change (with some examples), language change, and/or other cognitive change. They also were asked to provide other general comments relevant to the subject's social and psychological functioning. The NRAs perceived that 58% of the treatment women they rated improved in alertness by the end of the treatment program, 36% stayed about the same, and 6% regressed.

Among those whom the project staff perceived as having improved in alertness, the most frequent category of change cited was behavioral change. The types of behavioral changes cited included being more cooperative, having improved personality (usually being "more pleasant"), learning to ring the bell, having increased interest in personal appearance (e.g., wearing lipstick, having nails and hair done, wearing clean and dry clothes), being more talkative, and being more friendly. The language-related behavioral changes cited included being more talkative, being more open and honest, singing, using less nasty language, and screaming less.

The remainder of this section examines some of the common themes from the NRAs' assessments. These themes emerged from the NRAs' comments relevant to each patient's mobility, cognitive functioning, and incontinence, as well as from the section asking for anecdotes and insights the NRAs thought would be interesting and useful to case study analyses of women in the program.

REGULAR CAREGIVERS AND INCONTINENCE CARE

A recurrent theme was that the residents mistrusted the regular nursing staff caregivers, particularly with regard to incontinence care. Once a sense of trust in the NRAs was established, however, the results were often gratifying. A few excerpts from these assessments will illustrate.

1. Patient A began to trust more because she realized I wouldn't hurt her.

2. Patient B was very easy to relate to once she started to trust.
3. At first, Patient C wouldn't ring her bell. She was afraid the girl [regular caregiver] would yell at her.
4. Patient D was scared at first, but after we explained transferring and promised not to drop her, she really tried.

As noted in the first section of this chapter, the cognitive status of the treatment women in this program was quite low. Residents' perceptions of ill or substandard treatment by the regular caregivers may have been just that—perceptions, unsubstantiated by reality. However, the perception of mistrust was pervasive in certain facilities. This mistrust took different forms with different participants. Some women were afraid of being dropped during transfer from bed to toilet; others feared being embarrassed by the aides or publicly humiliated about their incontinence.

Some treatment women had bladder control but because of ambulation problems they needed someone to take them to the bathroom. Some of these women complained that aides were not there when needed, that the women would ring the bell or call and no one would come. An alternative complaint of some treatment women was that aides would put them on the toilet, leave, and not come back for as long as 40 minutes at a time. Residents' fear (whether justified or not) of being left on the toilet could conceivably generate some incontinence as an alternative to toileting.

Three brief case studies will illustrate how staff perception that one is too difficult to transport to the toilet can influence not only resident care but also the outlook and behavior of residents.

Case 1
According to the project staff, the regular nursing aides had Patient E believing she was too fat to handle. This was apparently why she would just wet herself rather than ask for the toilet. One evening at supper, Patient E wouldn't eat. She told the NRA she was too fat and wanted to diet. The staff liked this particular resident; they just didn't like handling her because of her weight.

Case 2
Patient F suffered from Parkinson's disease and arthritis. She did not have enough strength in her hands at the onset of the program to summon the aides with a regular bell or buzzer. The director of nurses at the facility did not have this woman on the original list of potential candidates for the behavior therapy program because "she is constantly wet." However, Patient F was included in the study and randomly assigned to the treatment group.

The project staff found that Patient F could hold her urine; in fact, she normally would void only once on the 7 A.M. to 3 P.M. shift and could usually tell the NRAs in advance. This individual told the project staff that the aides had told her she was easier to clean wet in the bed than to take to the toilet. Though physically impaired, this woman was mentally alert enough to be embarrassed about wetting herself. She responded well to the behavior therapy—both to the frequent opportunities to toilet inherent in the program and to the respect and individualized care provided by the project staff. Patient F greatly appreciated not being constantly wet.

Case 3

Patient G had been using a bedpan for over 2 years prior to the implementation of the behavior therapy program. In that time, she had not been taken to the bathroom to toilet. Patient G was very pleased to find she could stand and later take a few steps. She learned to hold her urine for longer periods of time and trusted the NRAs not to drop her. According to the project staff, this individual actually began looking forward to going to the toilet. She also became more talkative. During the 6-month follow-up phase of our study, the data collector found that the aides did not take Patient G to the bathroom. She was once again using the bedpan.

RELATIONSHIP BETWEEN PROJECT PATIENTS AND PROJECT STAFF

As noted, many of the treatment women were severely cognitively impaired. It was not unusual to have women who, particularly at the outset, could not remember from hour to hour who the NRA was, why the NRA was there, or what the protocol was. In some cases, the project staff perceived that a patient was motivated to cooperate but simply could not remember from hour to hour what she was expected to do. The project staff had both the time and the patience to work with these women to maximize their success with the program.

The trust that developed between the participants and the project staff enabled some participants to confide in the NRAs about their personal problems, including their previous experiences with their incontinence. Some were alert enough to be embarrassed by their incontinence. One participant was quoted as saying, "I know people took notice to my wet pants. I didn't like it." Other participants feared the anticipated repercussions (verbal scolding leading to humiliation at the least) from regular nursing home aides when they were found wet. These women were relieved to discover that the project staff would not be angry if they were wet. Perhaps the participants' ability to relax concerning their incontinence enabled them to improve. It was said about one woman in the study, "She'd strive to please us because we didn't verbally abuse her or add to her shame when we cleaned her."

The other side of this picture comes from regular nursing home aides. According to the regular aides, some individuals in long-term care wet simply "out of spite." It was suggested that some women use their incontinence to their advantage, to "pay back" aides not solicitous enough to suit them.

Whatever the case, the people who conducted the follow-ups in these homes reported regression of many participants after the treatment period was completed. Some participants remembered the project staff when they returned to do follow-up, but the attitudes, personalities, and sometimes the incontinence patterns of the women in the study were not as good during follow-up as they had been at the end of the treatment period.

IMPORTANCE OF SOCIAL REINFORCEMENT

Why did three-quarters of the treatment women improve their continence as a result of this prompted toileting program? The most frequent answer of the project staff was that the participants loved the social reinforcement (attention) they got when they were dry. A separate paper that examines patient behavioral response to this treatment therapy (Kaltreider et al. 1990) suggests that an important contributor to the improvement was the increased number of self-initiated requests to toilet made by the treatment women. Another very important contributor was the social reinforcement the treatment women received when they were dry. We believe that the participants learned early in the treatment period to associate the appearance of the NRA with something pleasant—that is, the social reinforcement. They would therefore request toileting in the hope that they could remain dry and receive the "reward" (conversation and extra time spent with them).

Some direct quotes from the NRA assessment forms suggest strongly that the social reinforcement (i.e., the extra time and attention given a resident when she was dry on the hourly checks) was important to the program's overall outcome.

1. Patient H picked up on the positive interaction [the 5 minutes of reinforcement] right away and put it to use.

2. Patient I was unsure of us at first, but she liked it when she wasn't wet because then she had someone to do things with or just someone to talk to.
3. Patient J was easy to get along with. She craved attention and responded very well to the time I spent with her when she was dry.
4. Patient K loved having someone share their time with her.
5. Patient L loved the special attention. She became more active [more time out of her room visiting and going to more activities].
6. I am not sure if Patient M benefited as much from the program itself [the prompting and toileting] as she did from just having company to talk to every hour.

One seemingly obvious key to the "success" of this program was that the project staff had no responsibilities except the treatment program. They could focus all of their efforts on this one particular aspect of the residents' lives. They were paid better than the average nursing home aide in the participating facilities. In addition, the research team tried to make the NRAs feel worthwhile about what they were doing and to instill in them a sense that they really could help these women reduce their incontinence. Furthermore, the project staff had the "luxury" (regular aides might say) of getting to know individual patients, of working with them as individuals, and of caring for them.

A good example of the payoff that could result from this individualized effort was a resident who was so "mean-spirited" at the outset of the program that she would spit on the NRAs. She would not get up out of her chair. After working with this woman for several weeks, the project staff uncovered a pleasant personality. The regular nursing aides in the home were amazed at the success the NRAs had with her. Initially, some aides had discouraged the research team from trying to work with this woman because she was "impossible." Her family also was amazed at the progress she made during the treatment program. This kind of emotional success is extremely hard to measure, but it existed and needs to be recognized.

In conclusion, the women who received the behavior therapy program decreased their urinary incontinence. As with many behavioral intervention programs, it is difficult to explain the process by which the program's effects are achieved. The most straightforward and simplest explanation is that social reinforcement resulted in the changes observed by the NRAs. It may well be that the social reinforcement had its effect because the behavioral interactions built trust and the residents formed a warm and trusting relationship with the NRAs. Indeed, one would hope that the social reinforcement program would produce this relationship change. Regardless of how the process by which the behavioral program produced its results is explained, it is important to remember that it was the behavior (prompting and social reinforcement) of the NRAs that was the independent variable in the study. Practitioners could implement the behavioral intervention program and expect to produce the practical, observed results of this study.

Participants were very old, mostly impaired, dependent elderly women in seven central Pennsylvania nursing homes. These women, many of whom had multiple physical, cognitive, and functional impairments, learned to request assistance for toileting, and if the assistance was provided when requested, the majority reduced their incontinence during the training period. They also retained much of their improvement in continence beyond the training period during a 6-month follow-up period.

IMPLICATIONS FOR PATIENTS AND HEALTH CARE PROVIDERS

According to the NRAs' assessments, this behavior therapy program had a positive effect on the social-psychological functioning levels of many of the participants. The improvements could not be documented by the participants' pretest and posttest scores on the psychological instruments administered, but several alternative factors that may have affected those results have been discussed.

We believe our findings are important for policymakers, health administrators, physicians, and nurses and for all those who work with extremely old, institutionalized patients. Men and women in the United States are reaching 65 years of age in greater numbers and proportions than they did before 1980. As the proportion of elderly people in the population has increased, the number of nursing homes has also increased (National Center for Health Statistics 1981). The age distribution of nursing home residents is changing: in 1977 those 85 and older comprised 40% of the elderly residents—up from 31% in 1964 (National Center for Health Statistics 1981). As the proportion of frail elderly persons increases, the responsibility of caring for those who are ill has shifted from families and friends to hospitals and long-term-care institutions, depending on whether the elderly patients have acute or chronic illnesses. This study focused on institutionalized female patients. This clinical trial empirically documented that institutionalized, female elderly can learn to ask for toileting help and that their continence status can be improved. This study also documented impressionistically that a behavior therapy program can improve the psychological status of incontinent residents in long-term care. These findings have important implications for health care providers and for policymakers.

REFERENCES

Bandura A: Social Learning Theory. Englewood Cliffs, NJ, Prentice-Hall, 1977

Brazda JF: Washington report. The Nation's Health 13:3, 1983

Brocklehurst JC, Griffith L, Fry J: The prevalence and symptomatology of urinary infection in an aged population. Gerontology Clinic (Basel) 10:242–253, 1968

Burgio KL, Burgio LD: Behavior therapies for urinary incontinence in the elderly. Clin Geriatr Med 2:809–827, 1986

Craighead WE, Kazdin AE, Mahoney MJ: Behavior Modification: Principles, Issues, and Applications, 2nd Edition. Boston, MA, Houghton Mifflin, 1981

Diokno AC: Urinary incontinence in the elderly, in The Practice of Geriatrics. Edited by Calkins E, Davis PJ, Ford AB. Philadelphia, PA, WB Saunders, 1986, pp 358–369

Duprey HJ: Self-representation of general psychological well-being of American adults. Paper presented at American Public Health Association Meeting, Los Angeles, CA, October 1978

Folstein MF, Folstein SE, McHugh PR: Mini-Mental State: a practical method for grading the cognitive state of patients for the clinician. J Psychiatr Res 12:189–198, 1975

Freeman RM, Baxby K: Hypnotherapy for incontinence caused by the unstable detrusor. Br Med J 284:1831–1834, 1982

Harris T: Aging in the eighties: prevalence and impact of urinary problems in individuals age 65 years and over. (Advance Data No 121). National Center for Health Statistics, U.S. Public Health Service, 1986

Hu TW: The economic impact of urinary incontinence, in Urinary Incontinence in the Elderly, Clinics in Geriatric Medicine. Edited by Ouslander J. Philadelphia, PA, WB Saunders, 1986, pp 673–688

Hu TW, Igou J, Yu L, et al: Cost effectiveness of treating urinary incontinent elderly—a bladder training program in nursing homes. University Park, PA, Institute for Policy Research and Evaluation, Pennsylvania State University, 1984

Hu TW, Igou JF, Kaltreider DL, et al: A clinical trial of a behavioral therapy to reduce urinary incontinence in nursing homes: outcome and implications. JAMA 261:2656–2662, 1989

Kaltreider DL, Hu TW, Igou JF, et al: Can reminders curb incontinence? prompting elders to void is a simple behavioral approach to incontinence. Geriatr Nursing 11:17–19, 1990

Mitteness LS, Wood SJ: Folk concepts of incontinence and social responses to the incontinent elderly. Paper presented at the 36th annual meeting of the Gerontological Society of America, San Francisco, CA, November 1983

National Center for Health Statistics: Basic data on depressive symptomatology, United States, 1974–75. Vital and Health Statistics series 11, no 216 (DHEW Publ No PHS-80-1666). Washington, DC, U.S. Government Printing Office, 1980

National Center for Health Statistics: Characteristics of nursing home residents, health status, and care received: National Nursing Home Survey, United States, May–December 1977. Vital and Health Statistics series 13, no 51 (DHHS Publ No PHS-81-1712). Washington, DC, U.S. Government Printing Office, 1981

Ory MG, Wyman T, Yu LC: Psychosocial factors in urinary incontinence, in Urinary Incontinence in the Elderly, Clinics in Geriatric Medicine. Edited by Ouslander J. Philadelphia, PA, WB Saunders, 1986, pp 657–672

Ouslander JG, Kane RL: The cost of urinary incontinence in nursing home patients. Med Care 22:69–79, 1983

Ouslander JG, Ulman GC, Urman H, et al: Incontinence among nursing home patients: clinical and functional correlates. J Am Geriatr Soc 35(4):324–330, 1987

Parker L, Whitehead W: Treatment of urinary and fecal incontinence in children, in Behavioral Pediatrics: Research and Practice. Edited by Russo DC, Varni JW. New York, Plenum, 1982, pp 143–174

Radloff LS: The CES-D scale: a self-report depression scale for research in the general population. Applied Psychological Measurement 1:385–401, 1977

Resnick NM, Yalla SV: Management of urinary incontinence in the elderly. N Engl J Med 312:827–835, 1985

Schnelle JF: Management of geriatric incontinence in nursing homes. J Appl Behav Anal 16:235–241, 1983

Spiro L: Bladder training for the incontinent patient. Journal of Gerontological Nursing 4:28–35, 1978

U.S. Health Resources Administration: A concurrent validation study of the NCHS general well-being schedule. Vital and Health Statistics series 2, No 73 (DHEW Publ No HRA-78-1347). Washington, DC, U.S. Government Printing Office, 1977

Weiss IK, Nagel CL, Aronson MK: Applicability of depression scales to the old old person. J Am Geriatr Soc 34(3):215–218, 1986

Wells T: Social and psychological implications of incontinence, in Urology in the Elderly. Edited by Brocklehurst JC. New York, Churchill Livingstone, 1984, pp 107–126

Willington FL: Incontinence—psychological and psychogenic aspects. Nursing Times 71(11):422–423, 1975

Wilson T: Incontinence of urine in the aged. Lancet 2:374–377, 1948

Yarnell JWG, St. Leger AS: The prevalence, severity, and factors associated with urinary incontinence in a random sample of the elderly. Age Ageing 8:81–84, 1979

Yu LC: Incontinence stress index: measuring psychological impact. Journal of Gerontological Nursing 13:7, 1825, 1986

Yu LC, Kaltreider DL: Stressed nurses dealing with incontinent patients. Journal of Gerontological Nursing 13:27–30, 1987

Yu LC, Hu TW, Kaltreider DL, et al: Profile of urinary incontinent elderly in long-term care institutions. J Am Geriatr Soc 38:433–439, 1990

Chapter Twelve

THE MAKING OF A GERIATRIC TEAM

Patricia A. Miller, Ed.M., O.T.R., and John A. Toner, Ed.D.

Dr. A., a psychiatrist on an inpatient unit, related an incident with a moderately demented patient, John, who consistently refused to follow directions from members of the unit staff. John remained in his room and had to be coaxed to leave his favorite chair to come to the dining room for meals and therapy. For the second consecutive day, Dr. A. was attempting to persuade John to join him for a walk, when a member of the housekeeping staff walked by and addressed the patient. "Flight #675 is leaving soon. Go with Dr. A.," she stated. Whereupon, John rose from his chair and proceeded to walk with Dr. A.

The housekeeping staff member used her knowledge of the patient's past history as an airline pilot to get him to move from his chair when she needed to clean his room. She had been doing this for 2 weeks, without the knowledge of any other staff members, prior to encountering Dr. A.'s problem in mobilizing John. "At that point, I learned the true value of interdisciplinary teamwork!" exclaimed Dr. A.

Although supporting delusions or nonreality-based behavior is usually contraindicated, this was the only approach to break the cycle of sedentary, isolated behavior in John. It was a starting point for activity engagement.

Why geriatric teamwork? Older patients may suffer from complex mental and/or physical chronic illnesses, which are often exacerbated by acute intercurrent conditions. In addition, the primary goal in the treatment of many older patients may not be the cure of disease but rather the attainment of an optimal quality of life, as defined by highly individualized functional and sociocultural criteria. To achieve comprehensive and coordinated care among multiple disciplines, teamwork is essential.

Successful clinical teamwork, like marriage and family life, depends on the presence of similar internalized values among team members. Going it alone compromises needs such as safety and comfort, as well as higher level needs affecting the quality of life. As with marriage and family life, however, the requisite knowledge and skills needed for successful teamwork are rarely taught to professionals in the course of their specialized education or in their subsequent clinical practice. Although statistics for failed marriages are readily available, those for malfunctioning or dismantled teams remain mysterious.

In this chapter, we will describe some of the basic concepts of team development, team management, and team maintenance as they were applied on a geriatric unit in a state hospital. After a brief literature review, we will describe methods for team development, with a major emphasis on goal setting for the unit. Next, we will present a problem-solving technique for improving care of a very difficult patient as an illustration of team management. Last, we will demonstrate team maintenance through a team process discussion that occurred on this geriatric team.

RELATED LITERATURE

Miller (1988) notes the dissatisfaction with the quality of problem solving at patient care meetings, where there is little or no shared treatment planning among disciplines: "These pro forma meetings have a negative impact on decision-making since the outcome is compromised by failure to identify significant dynamic issues and examine alternatives" (p. 123). Though skepticism regarding the value of teamwork may be symptomatic of malfunctioning teams, Rae-Grant and Marcuse (1968) warn readers that overvaluation of the importance of the team may lead to serious difficulties. These include 1) lack of critical monitoring of a team's goals and tasks, 2) diffusion of responsibility from one professional to the whole team, with the result that no one takes responsibility for the patient's care, and 3) a blurring of roles by teams so that the individual's expertise may be either weakened or underutilized.

A number of writers (Baldwin and Tsukuda 1984; Bennett and Miller 1987; DuCanis and Golin 1979; Sampson and Marthas 1981) have noted that tensions among disciplines regarding status, power, and territorial concerns are omnipresent and are often related to underlying personality conflicts. Despite these difficulties, these authors maintain that the requisite knowledge and skills for constructive interdisciplinary teamwork can be learned, thereby mitigating or eliminating the barriers to effective teamwork that affect quality care.

Many health professionals use the terms *multidisciplinary* and *interdisciplinary* interchangeably despite major differences in the philosophy and practice of each. Campbell (1983) and Baldwin and Tsukuda (1984) note that an interdisciplinary team approach emphasizes collaboration among professionals from diverse backgrounds who manage to share common goals and a joint responsibility for treatment outcome. In contrast, according to Takamura and colleagues (1979) and Bair (1983), members of a multidisciplinary team do not attend to interactional processes and generally tend to work independently.

Kane (1975) has observed that numerous definitions of teamwork exist that both reflect the biases of different authors and guide teams as to how they should function. We adhere to the following definition: "Teamwork is a special form of interactional interdependence between health care providers, who merge different, but complementary skills or viewpoints in the service of a patient in the solution of his or her health problem(s)" (Baldwin and Tsukuda 1984, p. 421).

Several authors (Baldwin and Tsukuda 1984; Campbell and Vivell 1983; DuCanis and Golin 1979; Rubin et al. 1975) point to the need for logical sequences in team development. These sequences progress from an initial period of goal setting and of defining and negotiating roles, through the development of a verbal and written communication system, to the ultimate establishment of a process for maintaining the team.

Other authors (Miller 1988; Sampson and Marthas 1981; Takamura 1983) stress the importance of understanding group dynamics to achieve productive team participation. Miller (1988) further notes that often too much emphasis is placed on maintaining the interpersonal needs of the team to the detriment of the team's tasks. She observes that it is only through the study of group dynamics that teams can be "taught the necessity of maintaining an appropriate balance between task functions and process study" (p. 126). It is important that team leaders and members consciously work on achieving this balance both to promote productive teamwork and to avoid becoming either too task or too process oriented. Bales (1958) elucidates this concept by describing the two types of behaviors that are needed for a group to work efficiently: task behavior and group maintenance behavior.

Takamura (1983) refers to the traditional medical model, which tends to appoint team leaders (most often physicians) on the basis of their possessing the highest rank within the hierarchical structure. In this model, the autocratic leadership style frequently prevails, with a consequent lessening of the importance of the viewpoints of the members. The essential message to the members is "Let me handle it. I know best" (Sampson and Marthas 1981, p. 207). Some of the effects of this leadership style upon team members are to create passive rather than active participation, to engender resentment and a lack of interest in problem solving, and to interfere with the members' capacities to function independently. In this regard, Sampson and Marthas (1981) observe that "a particular leadership style produces a corresponding membership style" (p. 209).

With respect to the interdisciplinary team approach, a democratic leadership style is the method of choice except in crisis situations, where "taking charge" meets an imminent need. Baldwin and Tsukuda (1984) describe the "emerging norm on many primary care teams which appears to be one of equal participation and responsibility on the part of team members" (p. 428). According to Takamura (1983), "When leadership roles and functions are not fixed with one member, ensuring the successful functioning of a team becomes the right and responsibility of every team member" (p. 68). Making the norm of equal participation and shared responsibility for the effectiveness of the team explicit rather than implicit provides a catalyst for interdisciplinary teamwork.

TEAM DEVELOPMENT: WILLARD PSYCHIATRIC CENTER

The interdisciplinary team training program described in this chapter is the outcome of 8 years of work devoted to the development of a durable, cost-effective method of linking and coordinating mental health services within the institutional setting. The program evolved, in part, from an educational philosophy that focuses on a participative model of self-education. The assumption is that the health care staff of an institution already have the technical skills required to function in their particular positions but need to enhance their understanding of how their roles on the team relate to those of others on the staff. In addition, a system by which the staff can work collaboratively to deliver effective treatment to patients is regarded as essential.

This concept was first applied in 1981 in an assessment training program involving teams at the Harlem Valley Psychiatric Center, a state mental hospital located one hour north of New York City (Toner

1982; Toner and Gurland 1983; Toner and Meyer 1988). Based on the results of this 2-year program, team training was evaluated systematically as part of an empirical study funded by the New York State Office of Mental Health and was applied to the development of the New York State Geriatric Psychiatry Fellowship Program.

The Geriatric Psychiatry Fellowship Program brings together the clinical resources of the Willard Psychiatric Center and the educational and clinical research resources of the Center for Geriatrics and Gerontology of Columbia University. The interdisciplinary team training program at the Willard Psychiatric Center exists within the structure of the fellowship program and is one of its central components.

The training was conducted on an experimental unit that was established by the Willard Psychiatric Center in consultation with the fellowship program faculty. It is an innovative, clinical model program of care for patients with dementia who are at risk for losing mobility. Team members of the unit volunteered to work there because they had a special interest in this type of patient population. With the support of the administration at Willard, team members were encouraged to develop an operations and procedures manual for the new unit. In this way, a structure and purpose for teamwork were established. Fellows were assigned to the unit during the second year of their fellowship training. The unit thus served as a laboratory for the fellows and the unit staff to be trained in the specific skills of team membership and leadership.

Setting Goals for the Patients and the Team

Goals define the aims and purpose of the team. Whether goals are mandated by the administration or developed primarily by the work group itself, members must identify them with clear, measurable end points to function effectively. Motivation for team participation increases when members have a sense of ownership of team goals. The establishment of team goals leads to behaviorally measurable accomplishments.

To foster team unity, team members wrote a core mission statement for the unit. This was accomplished by having the individual members of the unit write their perceptions of the team's purpose prior to attending the team meeting. A discussion of the individual viewpoints followed, and the following mission statement—the main goals of the unit—was developed by consensus:

A geriatric unit for patients with a diagnosis of dementia has been established to maintain and maximize the patient's level of functioning. By utilizing an innovative team approach to patient care and treatment, patients are kept safe from injury and free from restraints.

The patient's family members are provided support and assistance to cope with their relatives' progressive deterioration and are encouraged to participate in their treatment.

To determine whether the core mission statement was achievable, members of the team divided into three subgroups to write action goals. These goals began with a verb in order to be both measurable and attainable. Ten of the 23 goals developed by the team are included below.

1. Provide an environment that is safe and the least restrictive possible.
2. Reduce and/or eliminate chemical and physical restraints.
3. Develop goals that are appropriate for all geriatric patients, regardless of diagnosis, while individualizing goals for patients with specific needs.
4. Provide family support services.
5. Reduce stress and frustration in the environment.
6. Promote reality orientation.
7. Individualize patient care plans and goals recognizing the heterogeneity of the geriatric population.
8. Emphasize fall prevention with a multifaceted interdisciplinary program.
9. Establish geriatric educational opportunities for staff.
10. Develop consistent treatment interventions to be implemented by all three (day, evening, and night) shifts.

After the goals were written, team members discussed whether the goals were currently being attained and whether the members needed further definition, clarification, education, or problem solving to implement them to the fullest. The format for documenting the team's input was written on a flipchart during the team discussion and is included below (Table 12-1).

Establishing Priorities for Problem Solving

Between interdisciplinary team training sessions, team members were asked to prioritize the goals established according to their importance to the team's immediate or long-range interests. A high priority meant that issues related to attaining the specific goal should

Table 12–1. Clarification of team goals

Goal no.	In practice Yes	No	Remaining problems in achieving goals completely
1	X		Bathroom locks impede meeting the goal of providing the least restrictive environment. Safety problems exist when patient locks self in bathroom.
4		X	How, when, by whom, and in what context should family support services be provided?
5		X	Reducing stress and frustration needs to be defined and related to both patient and staff needs.
7	X day shift	X night shift	Understaffing creates problems of individualizing patient care plans to the fullest.

be addressed immediately, whereas a low priority signified that achievement of the particular goal was not a pressing need. This exercise, which also included having each participant circle team member(s)/discipline(s) responsible for fulfilling each goal, set the stage for further task differentiation and role definition and negotiation. A sample of the Goal Priority Form (Table 12-2) is included below.

Table 12–2. Goal Priority Form

Goal	Priority rating H M L	Reason for priority rating	In your opinion, which disciplines should be involved in carrying out goals on a regular basis? (Circle appropriate disciplines)
1. Provide safe and least restrictive environment			RN MD PA MHTA RT Admin OT SW MD/Psychiatrist PT
2. Reduce/eliminate chemical/physical restraints			RN MD PA MHTA RT Admin OT SW MD/Psychiatrist PT

Note. RN = nurse; MD = physician; PA = physician's assistant; MHTA = mental health therapy aide; RT = recreation therapist; Admin = administrator; OT = occupational therapist; SW = social worker; PT = physical therapist.

Results of Goal-Setting Exercise

As outsiders without administrative authority, the program's trainers wondered to what extent team members would pursue the team development process after the training was completed. All the goals and priorities for problem solving were developed and owned by the team. Carrying out any of the plans was strictly elective. Three months after completion of the team training sessions, the following changes were noted. While they may not seem particularly noteworthy to the casual reader, anyone who has struggled to make changes in a team setting can appreciate their significance.

1. The core mission statement was incorporated into the unit's Operations and Procedures Manual for the Specialized Geriatric Unit.
2. In response to goal 1 (provide an environment that is safe and the least restrictive possible), a requisition to place the dayroom television on a platform to eliminate hazardous wires and outlets was accomplished.
3. The Environmental Committee was notified of recommendations that would increase safety and be less restrictive—for example, to add dimmers on lights to reduce glare, to provide curtain rods without hooks to prevent danger when agitated patients tear curtains down, to rectify uneven heat on the unit (too cold or too hot), to supply rubber mats under lamps and dishes to prevent sliding, and to change bathroom locks for easier staff accessibility when patient is locked in the bathroom.
4. A team meeting was planned to solve problem with goals 4 and 12 (provide family support services and provide consultation services to prospective care providers). This was a consequence of plans to conditionally discharge four patients with dementia to family care homes. Special provisions were made to adapt the homes to accommodate wandering behavior and to provide special training to the prospective caregivers.
5. In response to goal 10 (develop consistent treatment interventions to be implemented by all three shifts), the unit changed the time of patient care meetings to enable the day and evening shifts to hold weekly patient care meetings together.

TEAM MANAGEMENT: SYSTEMATIC PROBLEM SOLVING (SPS)

The approach to problem solving we will describe is not new. What *is* unique is its application to geriatric practice. It can be used by educators, service providers, intra- and interdisciplinary teams, and family and self-help groups to identify and solve problems in a systematic and reasoned way while defusing emotions that hinder communication.

In stressful or crisis situations, decisions are often made prematurely, without the true nature of the problem being defined or alternative solutions being considered. To solve problems effectively, it is essential to understand the difference between problem solving and decision making.

The essence of problem solving is an appreciation of the fact that one is wrestling with the as yet unknown (Levenstein 1972b). "While problem-solving occurs when the alternative courses of action are unknown, decision-making is essentially a choice among known alternatives" (Levenstein 1972a, p. 61). Decision making, therefore, is one of the later steps in the problem-solving process, occurring after the problem has been defined and possible solutions have been explored.

The problem-solving process described herein includes six steps.

Step 1: Defining the problem. "A problem exists when a goal is unreachable or if there is a discrepancy between the way things are and the way things ought to be" (Center for Interdisciplinary Education in Allied Health 1980, p. 116). To define the problem accurately, it is necessary to ask as many questions as possible. Questions that begin with who, when, and where are useful in eliciting facts; questions that begin with what, how, or why are likely to be most effective in stimulating thinking about solutions (Levenstein 1972b, p. 365).

Step 2: Brainstorming solutions. Brainstorming, as defined in this instance, involves generating one idea from each participant while postponing any judgment as to its efficacy. Any suggestions regarding ways to solve the problem at hand are encouraged without discussion, criticism, or premature rejection of possible solutions. If the team members have more solutions to offer after each has an opportunity to speak once, the facilitator goes through the process again.

Step 3: Choosing a solution. All ideas generated in the brainstorming session are reviewed, and the possible solutions are discussed with all the individuals involved. The merits of each solution are evaluated in terms of three criteria: time, cost, and enthusiasm of the participants. The choice of which solutions to use is arrived at by group consensus.

211

Step 4: Planning ways to implement the solution(s). Delegation of responsibilities for carrying out one or more of the suggested solutions is essential before acting. Roles are defined and negotiated at this time, and commitments and tasks that members will undertake are recorded.

Step 5: Carrying out the plan. An appropriate time to carry out the plan is established, and the suggestions developed in steps 3 and 4 are put into practice. It should be noted that difficulties that impede progress toward a solution often arise while the plan is being carried out. In that case, members meet again to evaluate conflicts in resolving the problem.

Step 6: Evaluating the solution. Within an agreed on time, it is determined whether the plan of action is working. If it is not completely satisfactory to any one person involved and if modifications are indicated, the problem-solving steps are reintroduced. Ongoing support from the administration is vital to success.

A Patient Care Conference Using SPS

Patient Summary

Mrs. M., an 80-year-old white widowed woman with a diagnosis of primary degenerative dementia, Alzheimer's type, was transferred from a community hospital to the Willard Psychiatric Center 3 months prior to the team's SPS conference. She had also fractured her wrist. While in the community hospital, Mrs. M. became agitated, violent, and unmanageable.

The patient's son reported that Mrs. M. had become increasingly confused, forgetful, disoriented, and prone to aggressive episodes over the past 2 years. Prior to that time, there was no history of emotional problems, alcohol or substance abuse, or prior psychiatric treatment. She was a high school graduate and had been employed as a secretary for 20 years. Her son and her brother expressed the hope that Mrs. M. would improve sufficiently to allow her to return home, but they realized that a skilled nursing facility might be indicated.

On examination, Mrs. M. was moderately to severely demented. She was disoriented as to time and place and had impairments of memory for recent and remote events. Her insight and judgment were totally impaired. Wandering was frequent, and she required assistance in self-care activities with the exception of feeding. She was medically stable and had no physical problems requiring attention. Her affected wrist was functional. On admission to the unit, the patient was given thiothixene concentrate, 5 mg qid, and oxazepam, 15 mg po bid.

After the unit charge nurse presented the patient summary, the team members expressed specific complaints regarding the patient's behavior. Out of this process a team definition of the patient's problem evolved. This preceded the remaining steps of the SPS. All the problem-solving steps are included as developed by the team members although we have slightly paraphrased them.

Specific complaints of staff regarding the patient's behavior: Wanders, assaults reactively (when she is provoked verbally by other patients), undresses constantly, resists and disrupts bathing procedure, doesn't sit still long enough to eat meals, is incontinent of urine, shows little evidence of family support (few visits), occasionally bumps into things when walking with eyes closed.

I. *Defining the Problem*
"How might we reduce patient's disoriented, agitated, and disruptive behavior to promote a more manageable status on the unit while increasing her comfort and functional ability?"

II. *Brainstorming Solutions*

III. *Choosing Solutions*
and
IV. *Implementing Plans for Solutions*

1. Review medications and administer them 30–60 minutes before morning care.

1. *Physician* will change orders and *nursing* will administer medication at 6:30 A.M. (to decrease disruptiveness).

2. Increase environmental cues (pictures, signs) to promote orientation and reduce incontinence—for example, picture of toilet on bathroom door, picture of herself on bedroom door.

2. Not a unit responsibility. *Nurse* and *occupational therapist* will bring recommendations to hospital committee and report back to unit.

3. Reduce agitation and increase attention span; reduce sensory overload with more individualized attention.

3. One-to-one attention will be increased using unit quiet area. All unit staff involved; *recreation therapist* will coordinate effort.

4. Obtain eye consult to ascertain reasons for walking with eyes closed.

4. *Physician* will request eye consult.

213

5. Eat meals separately from other patients with one staff member to increase tolerance for sitting, eating, and engaging in an activity.

5. *Nursing* staff will seat patient at a separate table for 3–4 weeks and evaluate outcome.

6. Maintain log to determine how, when, and where incidents of assaultive behavior are precipitated.

6. Little enthusiasm by staff for this solution. *Nurse* and *occupational therapist* will consider at a later date, if necessary.

7. Check with family to determine eating and bathing habits prior to admission.

7. *Social worker* accepts responsibility. Will report findings to unit staff informally.

8. Promote orientation and reduce agitation by maintaining patient on this same unit. She has been transferred frequently.

8. All staff agree to work on stabilizing her environment on the unit.

V. Carrying out the plan was accomplished after the team training sessions during the trainers' absence.

VI. *Evaluating the Solutions*
Six weeks after the SPS patient conference, the team trainers elicited feedback from team members regarding Mrs. M.'s progress. According to several team members, Mrs. M. had improved. She was more alert (responding to single commands), walked with her eyes open, and was no longer incontinent. Agitation was reduced, and she was able to sit still long enough to eat her meals in the presence of other patients without being disruptive.

How did this occur? Upon initial questioning, some team members stated that they didn't do anything differently; Mrs. M. became accustomed to her new environment and that alone accounted for her improvement. Upon closer investigation, however, it appears that the following interventions based on brainstorming during the SPS conference may have accounted for some of her improvement:

1. The psychiatrist changed her medication from 5 mg thiothixene concentrate to 2 mg thiothixene capsule bid. The 15 mg oxazepam is continuing, po bid.
2. The social worker encouraged family members to visit more frequently, and they have responded positively. Mrs. M. seems to enjoy their visits and recognizes her son and her brother.

3. One-to-one attention by occupational and recreational therapist and social worker may have improved her orientation and attention span and elicited more appropriate social behavior.

TEAM MAINTENANCE

At the end of each team meeting (in the last 10–15 minutes), the leader facilitates a team process discussion by asking: "How was our meeting? Did we accomplish our goals? How could each of us have improved the meeting?" Team process discussions, as a norm for interdisciplinary teamwork, are a method for teams to monitor their own performance in a structured, supportive environment. Resistances to change, based on a repertoire of maladaptive defenses, are integral to malfunctioning teams and can be mitigated or eliminated by setting aside time for team process discussions.

Because formalized training in team development and management was new to this geriatric unit, one hour was devoted to determining team members' reactions to using SPS as a method for resolving team issues and patient care problems. Members knew that the team facilitators, as outsiders, would not be critical and could not be punitive in response to the members' reactions.

With the explicit norm of the group being the freedom to disagree and to avoid "group think" (Janis 1972), negative reactions surfaced quickly. A few examples follow:

"We don't have the luxury of brainstorming or problem solving."

"This is too time-consuming to use with every patient."

"The record-keeping method mandated by the state is very different from SPS, and therefore, the documentation can't be transferred to the required form."

"Problems are solved as they come up by one, two, or three people on a regular basis. We don't need team meetings."

"We can't suddenly change our schedules and include the evening shift in our patient care meetings. We have program plans set for weeks in advance."

Several team members then began to describe the ways in which they benefited from SPS.

"Our routine patient care meetings don't provide many brainstorming opportunities because of the speed we use to develop goals and treatment plans."

215

"We tend to repeat objectives in our routine meetings so that individualizing according to patients' needs is diminished."

"With SPS we were able to share our knowledge about psychogeriatrics and learn from each other."

"It was helpful to have the input from the mental health therapy aides. They usually do not attend patient care meetings unless a specific request is made."

"It may be useful to meet for SPS before problems become crises. For example, a meeting to discuss discharging our patients to family care homes would reduce the potential trauma to everyone involved."

Taking into account the difficulties of integrating SPS into already demanding schedules, the team came up with the following solutions for expanding opportunities for productive dialogue.

1. Include SPS methods (brainstorming) into weekly, routine, state-mandated patient care meetings.
2. Use SPS only with patients who are difficult to manage and are not benefiting from current treatment plans. Any team member can take the initiative for an SPS case conference as needed, or a designated time for SPS meetings—for example, every 4 or 6 weeks— could be allocated.
3. Use SPS for in-service training to achieve patient care goals while learning more about geriatrics.
4. Use SPS for achieving team goals, such as discharge planning of patients with dementia to family care homes. Education about how to ease the transition and resolve subsequent difficulties after the patient is living with a family requires planning. The social worker suggested the meeting and the psychiatrist suggested a date 5 weeks later, which the team agreed upon. The social worker and the occupational therapist negotiated facilitator and recorder roles for this particular meeting.
5. Two members suggested videotaping SPS at the next meeting and sending it to us to critique. This would provide initial supervision with these new team methods and would have potential use for training other hospital units in SPS. The members stated that their team had more open, trusting communication than other units in the hospital and that SPS serves to foster cohesiveness as members get to know each other's philosophies about care and specific interventions.
6. The member who originally stated that he could not change his program so that patient care meetings could be held in the afternoon to include the evening shift suggested that meetings with both shifts could commence in 2 months. This would allow time

for necessary administrative and programmatic changes. All team members agreed.

The facilitators warned the team that the path of least resistance was to maintain the status quo because of the reality of demanding schedules and people's natural resistance to change. Meetings are needed to formalize a mechanism for managing and maintaining the new components of the team's functioning. The team was left with the options to pursue these recommendations and to maintain the team trainers as resources via telephone, videotapes, and possible future visits until confidence and competence are achieved.

CONCLUSION

Interdisciplinary teamwork is vital if the multiple, complex needs of older persons are to be met in a comprehensive and cost-effective manner. Education in teamwork should not be considered elective for prospective or current health care professionals. Early collaborative experiences of students and clinicians from various disciplines act as a catalyst for internalizing a commitment to cooperative work.

The requisite knowledge and skills for team development, management, and maintenance can be learned, along with group dynamics, to increase the effectiveness and efficiency of teams. Ongoing support and resources from administration are needed to overcome the resistance to change inherent in every system.

We chose to highlight one example each of team development (goal setting), team management (SPS), and team maintenance (a process discussion) from our consultation experiences. We could not deal with relevant knowledge and skills related to role definition, role expectations, leadership, decision making, methods of communication, and conflict resolution in this chapter.

"The issue is clearly not one of team versus no team, but rather what kind of team, under what conditions, and for what purposes?" (Baldwin and Tsukuda 1984, p. 433). The prevalence of malfunctioning teams should not discourage geriatric practitioners from working collaboratively and seeking support for team training in their own work settings. The primary responsibility of each clinician is to his or her geriatric patient's optimal well-being. The only question is how this can best be accomplished.

REFERENCES

Baldwin D, Tsukuda R: Interdisciplinary teams, in Geriatric Medicine: Medical, Psychiatric and Pharmacological Topics, Vol II. Edited by Cassell C, Walsh J. New York, Springer-Verlag, 1984, pp 421–435

Bales R: Task roles and social roles in problem-solving, in Readings in Social Psychology, 3rd Edition. Edited by Macoby E, Newcomb T, Hartley E. New York, Holt, Rinehart & Winston, 1958, pp 437–447

Bair J: Programmatic treatment. Am J Occup Ther 37:11–13, 1983

Bennett R, Miller P: Interdisciplinary approach to graduate health sciences education in geriatrics and gerontology, in Handbook of Applied Gerontology. Edited by Lesnoff-Caravaglia G. New York, Human Sciences Press, 1987, pp 155–170

Campbell L, Vivell S (eds): Interdisciplinary Team Training for Primary Care in Geriatrics: An Educational Model for Program Development and Evaluation. Los Angeles, CA, Veterans Administration Medical Center, 1983

Center for Interdisciplinary Education in Allied Health: Health Systems Clerkship Study Guide and Resource Manual. Lexington, KY, University of Kentucky, 1980

DuCanis A, Golin A: The Interdisciplinary Health Care Team. Queenstown, MD, Aspen Publications, 1979

Janis I: Victims of Groupthink. Boston, MA, Houghton Mifflin, 1972

Kane R: Interprofessional Teamwork (Manpower Monograph No 8). Syracuse, NY, Syracuse University School of Social Work, 1975

Levenstein A: The art of decision-making, in Improving the Effectiveness of Hospital Management. Edited by Bennett A. New York, Metromedia Analearn Publishers, 1972a, pp 58–77

Levenstein A: Problem-solving through group action, in Improving the Effectiveness of Hospital Management. Edited by Bennett A. New York, Metromedia Analearn Publishers, 1972b, pp 355–372

Miller P: Teaching process: its importance in geriatric teamwork. Physical and Occupational Therapy in Geriatrics 6(3/4):121–130, 1988

Rae-Grant Q, Marcuse D: The hazards of teamwork. Am J Orthopsychiatry 38:4–8, 1968

Rubin I, Plovnick M, Fry R: Improving the Coordination of Care: A Program for Health Team Development. Cambridge, MA, Ballinger, 1975

Sampson E, Marthas M: Group Process for the Health Professions. New York, John Wiley, 1981

Takamura J: Team management: the issue of leadership in an interdisciplinary team, in Interdisciplinary Team Training for Primary Care in Geriatrics: An Educational Model for Program Development and Evaluation. Edited by Campbell L, Vivell S. Los Angeles, CA, Veterans Administration Medical Center, 1983, pp 68–69

Takamura J, Bermosk L, Stringfellow L: Health Team Development. Honolulu, HI, University of Hawaii, John A. Burns School of Medicine, 1979

Toner J: Interdisciplinary treatment training: a training program in geriatric assessment for health care providers, in The Personalized Care Model for the Elderly, 2nd Edition. Edited by Nicholson C, Nicholson J. New York, Nicholsen & Nicholson, Inc., 1982, pp 25–37

Toner J, Gurland B: Interdisciplinary team training for geriatric health care providers (abstract). Gerontologist 23:191, 1983

Toner J, Meyer E: Multidisciplinary team training in the management of dementia: a stress management program for geriatric staff and family caregivers, in Alzheimer's Disease and Related Disorders: Psychosocial Issues for the Patient, Family, Staff, and Community. Edited by Mayeux R, Gurland B, Barrett V, et al. Springfield, IL, Charles C Thomas, 1988, pp 81–102

LONG-TERM PSYCHOTHERAPEUTIC TREATMENTS

Chapter Thirteen

GROUP PSYCHOTHERAPY IN LATER LIFE

Sanford I. Finkel, M.D.

WHY USE GROUP THERAPY FOR OLDER PEOPLE?

Group therapy for the elderly, as defined by Burnside (1978b), designates only groups that are conducted both with older people who have significant emotional and/or mental problems and by professionals with special training in psychiatry or psychology. Berger and Berger (1973) define group psychotherapy as a treatment in which acknowledged patients voluntarily attend meetings with an acknowledged therapist at regularly scheduled intervals in order to express, evoke, accept, and work through various aspects of the patient's functioning to develop the patient's healthier and more satisfying potentials. Yalom (1975) states that the group provides a beneficial and controlled life experience by establishing relationships with the leader or interaction with group members, or both, together with some clarification of one's motives and those of others in the interaction.

Tross and Blum (1988) believe that group psychotherapy is the treatment of choice for older individuals with problems of social isolation, a sense of inadequacy, and a lack of meaningful interpersonal interactions. The group provides a forum for feedback about individual problems that allows for consensual validation and often cognitive alternatives. Further, if the patient demonstrates sufficient ego strength and motivation, the group can help the individual work through unresolved conflicts—sometimes those of long standing. Thus, group psychotherapy can address not only age-specific issues but also ongoing characterological problems.

Butler and Lewis (1982) found that intergenerational group psychotherapy resulted in an amelioration of suffering, the overcoming of disability, opportunities for new experiences of intimacy and self-fulfillment, and the opportunity to verbalize feelings.

Yalom (1975) describes 11 factors that are crucial to change in groups; Yost and Corbishly (1985) highlight 5 of these factors. Two of the most important are socialization and group cohesiveness. With many older people experiencing a significant reduction in number of meaningful relationships, membership in a group can decrease social isolation and impart an opportunity for identity and belonging. Further, the group offers opportunities to vitalize and maintain social skills, which in turn can lead to the application of those skills to new situations and human contact. The group also provides opportunities for receiving and giving affection and nurturance.

The other three integral factors Yalom identifies are universality, instillment of hope, and imparting of knowledge. The opportunity to see that one is not alone in one's plight can, in and of itself, allay anxiety. Knowing that others confront similar situations and especially seeing how others cope or fail to cope with such circumstances are often useful for finding new directions. The feeling of importance gained from being helpful to others and needed is a special feature of group therapy that has few parallels in individual therapy.

Verwoerdt (1976) emphasizes that group experiences result in an appreciation for the value of external sources of satisfaction as well as for the effectiveness of reality testing. Thus, such topics as "the good old days," religion, societal attitudes, and complaints about others can be discussed in the group with a full range of emotions expressed or vented.

Klein et al. (1966) emphasize the importance of having older people participate in an active way. Some of the programs available for older people have infantilized them, planning for the older persons rather than involving the older persons in planning for themselves.

Wolff (1970) points out that anxiety decreases in group therapy. Further, transference to one or more members is easy to achieve because of the variety of choices, and meaningful discussions are possible because a common goal or interest can be found with less effort. Wolff elaborates that the elderly patient develops a transference to the therapist as a peer-inspiring figure whose presence provides a feeling of protection for him. Acceptance by the group is also important to a patient. Further, the patient's feelings of difference and isolation decrease because the patient is sharing problems with others.

Lothstein (1988) believes that patients show concern and caring for each other. Patients whom she studied had a desire and a capacity to enhance object relationships that were meaningful and sustaining.

Older people frequently learn from each other as well as from the therapists, and often the person who gives the most also benefits the most in the process.

The economic aspect of group therapy is also important: mainly, it costs less than individual therapy. It also takes less in terms of professional resources in this practice area where, in spite of increasing numbers, there is still a paucity of trained therapists. The goals for group therapy vary greatly, depending on the setting, the ego strengths of the members, the experiences and expertise of the therapists, and time constraints. In inpatient and nursing home settings, there is enhanced staff and patient morale. At times there is even prestige in belonging to the group, and patients/residents may request to join—and even insist on it.

In summary, group therapy offers the following special opportunities for older people:

1. To reestablish formerly well-functioning defenses and coping mechanisms via interactions with other group members as well as opportunities to give to others and to enhance one's sense of usefulness.
2. To establish a sense of identity as part of a social entity, with a resulting increased libidinal stimulation.
3. To become part of a family unit with a nurturing supportive system, which the patient would then translate to other environmental situations.
4. To resolve old conflicts via reflection, reminiscence, reenactment, resolution, and growth.
5. To enhance self-esteem by ameliorating a harsh super ego that lends itself toward shame.
6. To adapt to and accept losses that cannot be reversed without expending excessive energy.

WHAT'S DIFFERENT ABOUT ELDERLY PATIENTS IN GROUPS

Altholz and Doss (1973) describe patients in their older groups as having more patience. They are more tolerant of silence and of monopolists. There is a greater tendency toward trust of the group process and a belief that they will receive a turn if they wait. Often their patience exceeds that of the therapist. Competitive issues in general are not as widespread as they are with younger group members.

Goldfarb (1966) points out that "younger persons in group psychotherapy break, remake, test, and consolidate relationships with others. . . . Older people do not seem to go through this process in their groups, no matter what the interests or the skills of the therapist" (p. 12).

Touching is considered much more acceptable in group therapy for older people. Hugging, holding hands, and putting an arm around someone is considered less conflictual than it might be with younger age groups. The tactile sensation may fill a sensory need caused by diminished visual and auditory perception. It also satisfies a psychological need when fewer interpersonal resources are available to provide warmth and libidinal stimulation.

Finkel (1981) compares younger outpatients in group therapy with older ones. He finds that virtually all members have some impairment in interpersonal relationships as a result of long-standing conflicts. For most, there has been a recent loss or disappointment that has led them to seek psychotherapy. Moreover, whereas a 50/50 gender ratio is relatively easier to obtain in younger age groups, it becomes very difficult with an older population. Further, the 6-month dropout rate is almost 50% in Finkel's (1981) older group population, although this is significantly skewed by Chicago winters, trips to Florida and other warmer climates, and illness. On the other hand, those older patients who remain often continue for several years. At 3 years, 25% of younger age group patients remained whereas 30% of older age group patients remained. Thus, though elderly group members are more apt to terminate early, they are also more apt to become long-term patients. This emphasizes the high degree of variability and individuality among older people.

Older people form alliances much more quickly. Usually within one to three sessions, one knows whether there is a "fit." In younger age groups, this process may take 6 to 12 months or longer.

Meerloo (1955) underlines the real and immediate way in which the therapist for an older age group member must fulfill a need for an interpersonal relationship that otherwise may be missing in the person's life. He theorizes a decrease in libidinal and aggressive impulses, which results in a hunger for a relationship with an idealized object. Thus, the therapist functions as both a real object and a transference object. At times, this leads to significant difficulties in effecting a termination.

Because one of the criteria for being a group member is to have the capacity to verbalize and introspect, individuals with certain conditions are usually excluded. These include patients with severe dementia, severe hearing impairment, and acute psychosis. The first two conditions are much more apt to occur with older age groups.

REVIEW OF THE LITERATURE

Silver (1950) is generally credited with publishing the first paper on group psychotherapy with older people. He conducted his work with 17 inpatient females between the ages of 70 and 80, all of whom had a diagnosis of senile psychosis. He stated that the group psychotherapy resulted in improved morale for both patients and nurses. Schwartz and Goodman (1952) conducted group psychotherapy with 19 obese, elderly outpatient diabetics. Thirteen of them lost a significant amount of weight, and two were able to discontinue insulin. Linden (1953, 1954, 1955) treated a group of senile female patients with intensive group therapy over a period of 2 years. Of those, 45% were ready to leave the hospital after an average of 54 hours of group therapy. Two-thirds of these were able to resume their customary activities. In the control group, consisting of patients not treated in groups, only 13% were able to leave. It should be pointed out, however, that the criteria for acceptance into the group resulted in a skew toward highly functioning patients. Didactic talks, good-natured sarcasm, and individual questioning were among Linden's therapeutic techniques. His descriptions on transference and dual leadership are classic and are described later in this chapter.

Wolff (1963, 1970) carefully chose 110 older hospitalized patients. Of those in group therapy, 50% were discharged within one year, as compared with 18% for the control group. Wolff viewed group therapy as a treatment of choice for the elderly patient because it is "less alarming." He emphasized that acceptance by the group is more important than acceptance by the individual. Wolff, as have others from inpatient settings, emphasized the importance of a supportive rather than an insight-oriented approach, believing that "the development of insight for older individuals is frequently not only impossible, but also undesirable." Others would strongly object to Wolff's conclusion and firmly believe in the value of insight (Grotjahn 1955; Lothstein 1988).

Others who studied the effects of group psychotherapy with the institutionalized aged in the 1950s and 1960s include Benaim (1957), Feil (1967), Liedermann et al. (1967), Lowy (1967), Rechtschaffen (1959), Ross (1959b), Schwartz and Goodman (1952), Shere (1964), Wolk and Goldfarb (1967), and Zimberg (1969).

The 1970s saw a surge in the amount of literature on group work with elderly people. These articles have contributed significantly to the application and understanding of group psychotherapy. Experiential and clinical experiences elaborate that group psychotherapy is effective in a variety of settings (Altholz and Doss 1973; Burnside 1978a; Butler and Lewis 1982; Cohen 1973; Conrad 1974; Finkel and Fillmore 1971; Goldfarb 1972; Rosin 1975).

In the past dozen years, innovative and comprehensive use of group psychotherapy has been described by Berkman (1978), Blum and Tross (1980), Burnside (1978b), Gallagher (1981), Hartford (1980), Killiffer et al. (1984), Levine and Poston (1980), Myers (1984), Parham et al. (1982), Saul (1983), White and Weiner (1986), Yesavage and Karasu (1983). Tross and Blum (1988) outlined the basic approaches to group psychotherapy in late life as insight-oriented, supportive, or cognitive-behavioral (Beck and Rush 1978; Beck et al. 1979; Gallagher and Thompson 1982b).

For insight-oriented group psychotherapy, the pioneer was clearly Linden (1953, 1954, 1955, 1957). Linden did emphasize structured methods at the onset in dealing with his state hospital elderly population. However, he used his role as therapist to establish a positive transference to an omnipotent parent to build group cohesion. He encouraged interpretation, the evolution of multiple transferences, and free association. It was Linden who introduced the use of male and female cotherapists as parental transference stimuli, sexual models, and models for opposite-sex object choice. Thus, Linden combined psychoanalytic practice with directive techniques to address his specific population.

Grotjahn (1955, 1978) stressed the value of group therapy in late life, with special emphasis on nursing home populations, where individuals need affective and cognitive stimulation. Grotjahn believed that the patient's potential for transference interpretation increases with age.

Krasner (1959, 1977) was one of the first to conduct analytically oriented outpatient group psychotherapy. His principles include using a nonauthoritarian approach; making no attempt to manipulate the environment or to place restrictions on the patients' reactions in group session; activating transference relationships; providing an accepting attitude; focusing and interpreting resistances; interpreting the transference phenomenon; providing insights that could help the group members achieve understanding of their thoughts and feelings about their current and past experiences; using this understanding to change present behavior to achieve greater freedom from conflictual pressures; and establishing and experiencing new values and

228

experiences within the group, which may then be utilized in outside situations. In this way, there can be a working through of early developmental conflicts.

Berland and Poggi (1979) began a supportive psychotherapy group for residents of a private retirement home. At the urging of the patients, the approach shifted from supportive to insight-oriented. Berland and Poggi discovered that older people wanted to change, had the capacity to form deep relationships with others, did not have significant cognitive deficits, and were able to abstract. They concluded that countertransference might be the primary reason that insight-oriented group therapy was not used more often.

Countertransference problems toward elderly persons have interfered with appropriate psychotherapy for the elderly from the time of Freud, who stated: "It [the psychoanalytic method] fails with people who are very advanced in years, because, owing to the accumulation of material in them, it would take up so much time that by the end of the treatment they would have reached a period of life in which value is no longer attached to nervous health" (Freud 1898, p. 282). Baker (1985) used Levinson et al.'s (1978) conceptual framework of developmental tasks and determined that the use of group and individual transferences resulted in substantial changes and growth.

In contrast with insight-oriented psychotherapy, supportive group therapy has been used to deal with specific age-related changes, which require adaptation as well as increasing comfort with dependency needs. Life review and reminiscence therapy has been shown to be superior to traditional psychotherapy with psychotic elderly inpatients (Lesser et al. 1981).

Gallagher and Thompson (1982b) demonstrated that a variety of group psychotherapy approaches are helpful for older people and that a cognitive, behavioral approach has a longer lasting effect. Yost and Corbishly (1985) emphasized that cognitive therapy combats attitudes and behaviors that can lead to depression in late life. The recommended method involves mutual participation by patient and therapist and includes designing homework assignments. This decreases dependency and compliance by the older person and increases a sense of control. In this highly structured therapy, specific and limited goals are set. Assignments focus on a single therapeutic principle at a time and often use behavioral techniques that require the patient to increase activity levels between sessions. This model also uses a great deal of questioning and includes lectures and discussions.

In spite of the substantial increase in the number of articles about group therapy with elderly patients, there remains a paucity of valid research data. Much of the literature contains clinical or anecdotal conclusions based on the therapists' perceptions. Some of the controlled studies involved comparisons of approaches. Steuer et al. (1982, 1984) compared the outcomes of psychodynamically oriented group therapy with those of cognitive-behavioral group therapy and concluded that both were useful, although the cognitive-behavioral group scored significantly higher on the Beck Depression Inventory (Beck et al. 1961).

STARTING A GROUP

Inception of a new group takes considerable time and energy. It represents a major commitment from patient and therapist alike. It must be entered into only with substantial discussion, including a careful explanation by the therapist to the patient of the potential rewards, shortcomings, and mutual obligations. All too often, groups are formed with minimal forethought, resulting in premature departure of members and early collapse of the group.

It is preferable to have a comprehensive diagnostic evaluation, preferably by both therapists (assuming there is dual leadership), with careful consideration given to the specific goals of the group and of the other potential members.

Hartford (1980) notes that when patients enter a group, their goals can be classified as

1. Conscious goals, which are compatible with the goals suggested by the leader
2. Conscious goals, which the patient is aware of but may not express within the group or to others—e.g., being with one's friends or with the group leader
3. Unconscious goals—e.g., gaining affection or personal gratification, gaining power and control

Any member may bring to the group any or all three of these types of goals and behave accordingly.

Advanced preparation involves more than establishing a therapeutic contract between therapist and patient. In institutional settings, administrative problems may abound. It is critical to have administrative support to cut through complex issues related to scheduling conflicts, questions of responsibility regarding patients coming to and from meetings, competitive feelings of other staff regarding removal of patients from other activities, potential competitive feelings from attending physicians and other psychotherapists who are not part of

230

the group, and feelings from participants who have been left out of the group therapy process. In state hospital settings, it may also be difficult to obtain accurate information about patients' histories and clinical status (Bienenfeld 1988).

Finally, one must take into consideration transportation for outpatients, as well as the ability to accommodate members with physical impairments—e.g., those requiring wheelchairs. One must also attempt to anticipate potential absences, which could significantly limit the group's effectiveness.

LEADERSHIP

It is generally considered ideal for a leader to like older people and to be honest, gentle, and open with him- or herself about issues related to death, disability, sexuality, and dependency.

There is general agreement that the use of cotherapists has substantial advantages, including

1. The mutual support between therapists
2. The group reaction to the therapists, which can enhance parental transferences
3. The addition of a role model
4. A decreased stress among therapists, given that one can serve as observer to the other in the midst of a group process
5. The ability to check out perceptions and to plan jointly
6. The ability of one therapist to work through his or her own resistances with the assistance of the cotherapist

Altholz and Doss (1973) recommend two leaders—even if not of the same sex—to sustain the physical and mental level of energy and enthusiasm that is necessary to lead the group. Matorin and Zoubok (1988) indicate that the presence of two leaders allows for splitting and alternating roles. When one was supportive or tolerant or expressed anger, the other could maintain an interpretive posture and proceed to set limits and, occasionally, to confront disruptive behavior or avoidance. Moreover, the strain of dealing with affectively charged material—most specifically, issues such as loss, death, and fear of dying—became more tolerable when shared with a coleader.

Lothstein (1988) emphasized that age of the therapist made little difference, as compared with gender. Often male physicians and female nurses or social workers were cotherapists. In particular, he found that group members devalued female group leaders, calling them by their first names, whereas they called the males (usually physicians) by the term *doctor*. Such situations demand an excellent communication between cotherapists to assist in a higher level of comfort and therapeutic efficacy.

MEMBERSHIP

The ideal number for a group is between 5 and 8 patient members, although between 4 and 12 may be considered acceptable. It is critical to have variety to provide a stimulus among group members. Although aging problems must have some commonality, there also needs to be some heterogeneity of problems. The size of the group must be large enough to contain variety, yet small enough to allow for personal involvement.

The criteria for membership must be established at the onset. For outpatient groups, it can be difficult to achieve balance. Advertisements in local newspapers often result in successful recruitment. However, certain patients with severe types of personality disorders—e.g., patients who are chronically isolated, schizoid individuals who are easily injured narcissistically, patients who cannot tolerate any anger or hostility, and patients who are sadistic and truly provocative to others—do not fit well into groups. Patients with severe hearing impairment, advanced dementia, incontinence, or acute and severe medical illness (pulmonary edema, angina, emphysema), or patients who are religious fanatics are also generally unacceptable as group members.

It is usually not advisable to mix former state-hospital patients with non-state-hospital patients. The same can be said about mixing demented individuals with nondemented ones. Frames of reference in commonality are very different between these individuals, and the leaders can expect tremendous ongoing resentment, hostility, rejection, and patient withdrawal from the group. At all times, it is important to maintain the respect of the individual patient and to protect that patient from potential harm.

THE SETTING

The setting must be comfortable, with special attention paid to noise levels, lighting, glare, comfortable furniture, handicapped accessibility, and temperature. Group therapy can be held in virtually any setting where such variables are controlled. The most common settings in the literature are within psychiatric hospitals, outpatient clinics, and nursing homes.

Another consideration is whether the group should be open or closed. Open groups are necessary in inpatient settings where patient flow is constant. On the other hand, outpatient group therapy may allow for long-term relationships to be formed in settings that minimize change in group composition. In fact, it is in such situations that the most profound change has been noted (Baker 1985).

The time allotment for the group session varies from 30 to 90 minutes, again depending on the setting and on the degree of functioning of the patients. In inpatient settings, the life of the group is interminable as the group repeatedly reconstitutes itself. Outpatient group psychotherapy may have a limited time frame, sometimes based on the period of training of the professional.

A real problem can occur when new members are added to a group. This may result in the aggression and withdrawal of someone who has unresolved issues regarding approval, sibling rivalry, or a sense of specialness.

Although Butler and Lewis (1982) described the advantages of age-integrated groups, the general feeling is that there should be a lower age limit to group therapy for elderly patients—e.g., mid-50s. Some believe that it is not a good idea to mix those in their 50s with those in their 90s inasmuch as most of the issues, conflicts, and themes are generally quite different.

THEMES AND GOALS

Group therapy with elderly patients abounds with common themes, regardless of setting or population:

1. *Social losses.* "My life changed when my husband passed away; now most of my friends are dead, too." "I lost my job, so now what?" "My children moved. That's why I am in the hospital." "Nobody loves you when you're old and gray."
2. *Independence versus dependence.* "I don't want anybody to take care of me. I can do fine myself." "I need help, but who's going to give it." "I want to give, but now I'm forced to receive. . . . It hurts . . . it hurts."
3. *Physical illness, pain, and sensory decrement.* "What good are you when you are in so much pain you can't conduct your life normally?" "How do I stop the discomfort of my arthritis?" (Finkel and Fillmore 1971, p. 195)

Other common themes include death, loneliness, the good old days, fear of memory loss, religion, historical events, helplessness and fear for the future, intergenerational conflicts, depression, treatment questions, sexuality and intimacy, and how to sustain a level of hopefulness.

Goals are varied and include providing narcissistic supplies to compensate symbolically for losses, halting regression, effectively reutilizing social skills, enhancing a sense of identity, providing useful information and information exchange, enhancing the sense of control over one's life—in part by facilitating giving and nurturing from each of the other, providing a safe forum for working through grief and other psychological issues, and providing support through times of crisis.

TECHNICAL ASPECTS OF BEING A GROUP PSYCHOTHERAPIST

The group psychotherapist must be a facilitator, clarifier, adviser, and interpreter for the group process. The relative degree of activity will depend on the therapist's own particular philosophy, defined role, technical skill, and professional stance and the context in which the group therapy occurs (Hartford 1980).

According to Yalom (1975), group maintenance and culture building are the two basic tasks of the group psychotherapist. Inasmuch as the members generally do not know each other prior to the inception of the group, the therapist acts as a "transitional object" and, at the onset, is the group's primary unifying source. It is not uncommon for group members to relate to the therapist and not to each other during the early phase of group psychotherapy.

Group maintenance also includes control of absenteeism and responsibility for maintaining an adequate number of members to sustain the group.

Mrs. Rosen missed three of the first five group therapy sessions. Though she presented several reasons, it was clear that she was anxious and fearful about exposing some of her problems to the group. When she arrived for the subsequent session, one of the women told her that at the time of her previous attendance, she (Mrs. Rosen) had made several interventions that were helpful to the woman. Mrs. Rosen was very moved by the impact she had had on this other woman and also realized that her absence at the previous group session interfered with the other woman's need to continue to discuss her issues with Mrs. Rosen. Her subsequent attendance was perfect except for extraordinary circumstances.

The leader must be on guard for scapegoating, absences, tardiness, and cliques.

> Mrs. Smith was a relatively passive, dependent, and depressed member in a group with several assertive participants. Whenever conflict arose and the assertive group members became anxious in their confrontations and challenges with each other, they would tend to focus on Mrs. Smith and her passivity and would become critical of her at these tense moments. The therapist intervened to point out this recurrent pattern, and this allowed the assertive group members to focus their own issues more effectively.

Culture building refers to the group establishing therapeutic norms that are consistent with the goals of therapy. These are established relatively early in the group and are difficult to change once established. Some groups place a great deal of emphasis on food and will bring in cookies, coffee, etc., for themselves or others. For other groups, food is brought in only on specific occasions, such as birthdays or a group member terminating. Yet for other groups, food is never brought in. The meaning of food to the individuals and to the group collectively can be explored. Often it has to do with a safe way of nurturing each other in a socially acceptable manner.

Yalom also describes the group leader as both a technical expert and a model-setting participant. The leader is asked questions on a whole variety of topics. Although it is often proper for him or her to respond directly, it is important for the leader to keep in mind the goal of having members interact with each other in a forthright, nondefensive, nonjudgmental manner.

> Mr. Bellow would often begin a session by asking the physician member of the group specific questions regarding medication—efficacy, side effects, etc. He asked not only about his own medication but also about medication he knew others to be taking. The group generally tolerated his questions and acted courteously. The therapists pointed out to Mr. Bellow that, although the information was important in one sense, it also served to focus attention away from a number of other issues regarding feelings and conflicts and their resolution. Such matters are more difficult to discuss than "factual, scientific matters." With several such interventions, Mr. Bellow eventually came to talk about issues related to his fear of the future, problems with his family, and physical health problems.

Ideally, the patient also observes the interactions between the therapist and other group members and internalizes and emulates some of the group therapist's approaches. This, in turn, enhances the patient's empathy and ability to give and receive.

The norm in group therapy for elderly patients is that the therapist be active although, as Bienenfeld (1988) points out, the meaning of active is rarely defined. Elderly people—even in chronic care institutions—need not be considered incapable of insight or self-examination. As Lothstein (1988) points out, an overly active leader will limit growth of the group and make it pathologically dependent on its leader. On the other hand, a silent and distant leader runs the risk of losing the group through a high dropout rate. Sakauye (1979) and Riley and Carr (1989) emphasize a relatively "inactive" approach, in which a nonstructured stance emphasizes the importance of recognizing the older person's ability to define his or her own perspectives on this stage of life, particularly when these perspectives conflict with the therapist's expectations. A therapist must feel comfortable with a slow pace and gradual movement while at the same time not providing excessive support and sympathy, which encourages dependency and regression.

The group therapist is also a link with the real world, sometimes one of just a few social contacts, a friend, or a model of social skills for how to give affection and reinforcement. The therapist may also bear the brunt of any negative feelings that the patient may feel toward his or her own children (Yost and Corbishly 1985).

OTHER ISSUES

Lothstein (1988) indicates that older patients in a group show concern and caring for each other. Issues of hostility, competitiveness, and aggression, which are often present in beginning groups of younger adults, are virtually absent in older age groups. She hypothesizes that this results from an expressed desire to seek out object relationships that are meaningful and sustaining. As the group progresses into its second year, progressive and competitive issues can emerge as people feel more comfortable with their connections to other group members. The group members' altruism is not necessarily defensive but rather socially adapted and developmentally necessary in order to link members with important objects.

When Mrs. Bloom felt particularly needy, she would enter the group and immediately express anger at the group and all of its members for being "powerless and uninterested" in addressing her problems. The therapist frequently commented that although Mrs. Bloom would express such thoughts and feelings, what she really wanted was to be nurtured by the group and told how much they liked her and what a good person she was. After several such interventions, other group members became aware of this dynamic and would frequently intervene in a similar way with Mrs. Bloom when she entered into one of her rages. Several group members commented that this insight was valuable outside the group and that they had learned to look beneath the expressed anger of friends and relatives to the dependency longings and wishes for nurturance.

On an inpatient general psychiatry unit with an older adult group therapy program, Mrs. Thompson brought Mr. Anton to his first group session. She had told him how helpful the group would be and hoped that he would accompany her. Mrs. Thompson felt very good about introducing Mr. Anton into the system. It enhanced her self-esteem to be helpful. It also allowed her to have a special rapport with the therapist, who thanked her for her thoughtfulness and kindness to Mr. Anton.

Intergenerational anger may be a reflection of the rivalry and envy toward younger therapists—particularly younger female therapists onto whom group members may project neurotic and aggressive feelings.

Mrs. Kendall had a long-standing, ambivalent, conflictual relationship with a daughter who lived next door to her. She frequently felt that the daughter did not spend enough time with her and neglected her for the daughter's own gratifications and other responsibilities. When these feelings and conflicts were at the forefront, Mrs. Kendall would often come in and express anger to the young female social worker therapist in the group. "I know that you young women are interested in your own lives, your men, your work, and your good times. You don't have time to respect your elders." The therapists were able to help her see that some of the anger directed at the social worker was transferential and directly related to the emotional climate between her and her daughter.

Older people are not uncommonly anxious about becoming a group member. Many retain an attitude toward mental illness that was prevalent in their youth, and thus they often believe that someone who needs a therapist must be crazy (Finkel 1979–1980). Further, many older people have been taught to be seen and not heard and have difficulty sharing their innermost feelings. Thus, feelings of shame and fear may be generated at the prospect of talking about personal concerns. Even when members have a desire for close physical proximity, their sense of privacy may cause anxiety about their wish for such closeness. It also may make them reluctant to seek help.

237

Mrs. Sweed had a long history of independent functioning. However, in the past 2 years, this 77-year-old woman had had both a mastectomy and a colostomy for carcinomas. She also lost her husband and had to move from her home of 37 years. She had great difficulty adjusting to all her new dependency needs. She had come from an environment in which she was the oldest of nine children, and she was used to a great deal of responsibility with little in return. She had come into therapy on the referral of her internist because of uncontrolled tearfulness and a sense that she was all alone in the world.

She entered the group but had great difficulty talking about feelings and issues that had been paramount on her mind. Several of the group members attempted to engage her, but this reinforced her sense of shame regarding her dependency.

Issues of confidentiality must be addressed early in the group process. This is particularly true in hospitals and nursing homes, where privacy may be minimal. One approach is to assure the group members that all information shared with the group is strictly confidential. However, it is judicious to make one qualifying statement that if someone's life is in danger, this rule may need to be broken—but only under such extraordinary circumstances. It is common for staff members in nursing homes or hospitals to ask the group therapist for specific information. However, to get into such a pattern of reporting would not allow the patient to express negative feelings about the unit, certain staff members, etc., because of fears of retribution—however irrational such concerns may be.

Corey et al. (1982) discuss the process issue of confronting and probing. They emphasize that older people need support and encouragement more than they need confrontation, and that any such probing or confrontation must therefore be done gently and with caution. A group process must allow opportunities for social interaction and pleasure. Some groups have refreshments before or after the group meeting in order to encourage such interaction. Many older people are fearful of new relationships inasmuch as they have been traumatized by the loss of those close to them. The energy required to develop a relationship may be initially perceived more as a burden than as a potential reward.

Successful group therapy has been characterized by both the feeling of identification with a group in relation to a mutual problem and the presence of a positive relationship between the individual and the group leader (Wolff 1970). Wolff notes that in heterosexual groups, both men and women significantly improve their appearances after becoming group members.

Opportunities for transferential/countertransferential phenomena are vast. The therapist may be considered an idealized child or an omnipotent parent by somebody two or three times his or her age. The therapist must feel comfortable with being idealized while understanding the meaning of this phenomenon for a given patient.

Van der Kolk (1983) describes transference-oriented group psychotherapy as providing boundaries for certain patients while also providing a sense of continuity and of usefulness to others. He states that projective identification can be explored only in a group setting. With its acknowledgment comes a decrease in the sense of loneliness and isolation. Envy toward the younger therapist can be most safely explored in a group setting. A patient's mourning for lost prowess can take place after participants sense that they are all "in the same boat." In such a group, therefore, the focus is not on the negative transference but rather on narcissistic injuries. This transference-oriented approach allows themes of loss and death to emerge and permits group members to provide each other with real gratification, which would not have been possible in individual therapy.

The therapist must be on guard against overidentifying as well as against denying the patient's anxiety, pains, and conflictual issues. In the early phases of being a group psychotherapist, the therapist's relationship with the supervisor—as well as with the cotherapist—is critical for his or her own insight, development, growth, and effectiveness.

MacLennan (1988), in his overview of psychotherapy with older people, concludes that the training of older and younger group therapists should include an understanding of their attitudes toward aging and death, both their own and others', and must be adjusted to the age and experience of the trainees. Older therapists are much more immediately attuned to the problems of active elderly patients who are their contemporaries, and they are less likely to evoke role reversal transferences. In groups made up of relatives of the very old and disturbed, therapists may encounter the same problems and frustrations they experienced with their own aged parents. Whatever the situation, therapists need to guard against countertransferences resulting in their own unresolved conflicts about aging. Linden (1955) emphasizes the importance of therapists recognizing their own stereotypes about aging; these must be overcome if therapists are to help their elderly patients.

In spite of the paucity of hard research data, therapists and staff alike believe that group psychotherapy is an excellent modality for dealing with the conflicts and problems of late life. For many patients, it helps to reestablish a sense of usefulness and identity, and it markedly diminishes the sense of isolation. It allows for reflection on old conflicts, including intergenerational issues, with development of new insight and resolution. Individual members have an opportunity to reflect on how other patients work through—or don't work through—similar conflicts, both present and past. The overall impact of the group is to enhance self-esteem and to adapt and accept certain losses, while respecting each individual's ability to adapt, change, and find new solutions to life's challenges.

REFERENCES

Altholz J, Doss A: Outpatient group therapy with elderly persons. Gerontologist 13:101–106, 1973

Baker FM: Group psychotherapy with patients over 55: an adult development approach. J Geriatr Psychiatry 17:79–84, 1984

Beck AT, Rush AJ: Cognitive approaches to depression and suicide, in Cognitive Defects in the Development of Mental Illness. Edited by Serban C. New York, Brunner/Mazel, 1978, pp 235–258

Beck AT, Rush AJ, Shaw BF: Cognitive Therapy of Depression. New York, Guilford, 1979

Benaim D: Group psychotherapy within a geriatric unit: an experiment. Int J Psychiatry 3:123–128, 1957

Benitez-Bloc R: Including the active elderly in group psychotherapy, in Group Psychotherapies for the Elderly. Edited by MacLennan BW, Saul S, Weiner MB. Madison, CT, International Universities Press, 1988, pp 33–42

Berger LF, Berger MM: A holistic group approach to psychogeriatric outpatients. Int J Group Psychother 23(4):432–444, 1973

Berkman B: Mental health and the aging: a review of the literature for clinical social workers. Journal of Clinical Social Work 6:230–245, 1978

Berland DI, Poggi R: Expressive group psychotherapy with the aging. Int J Group Psychother 29:87–108, 1979

Bienenfeld D: Group psychotherapy with the elderly in the state hospital, in Group Psychotherapies for the Elderly. Edited by MacLennan BW, Saul S, Weiner MB. Madison, CT, International Universities Press, 1988, pp 177–188

Blum JE, Tross S: Psychodynamic treatment of the elderly: a review of issues in theory and practice, in Annual Review of Gerontology and Geriatrics. Edited by Eisdorfer C. New York, Springer, 1980, pp 204–237

Burnside IM: Principles from Yalom, in Working with the Elderly: Group Processes and Techniques. Edited by Burnside IM. North Scituate, MA, Duxbury Press, 1978a, pp 114–127

Burnside IM (ed): Working with the Elderly: Group Processes and Techniques. North Scituate, MA, Duxbury Press, 1978b

Busse EW, Blazer DG (eds): Geriatric Psychiatry. Washington, DC, American Psychiatric Press, 1989

Butler RN, Lewis MI: Aging and Mental Health: Positive Psychosocial and Biomedical Approaches. St. Louis, MO, CV Mosby, 1982, pp 329–332

Cath S: Psychoanalytic viewpoints on aging—an historical survey, in Research Planning and Action for the Elderly. Edited by Kent DP, Kastenbaum R, Sherwood S. New York, Behavioral Publications, pp 279–314

Cohen MG: Alternatives to institutions for the aged. Social Casework 54(8):447–452, 1973

Conrad WK: A group therapy program with older adults in a high-risk neighborhood setting. Int J Group Psychother 24:358–360, 1974

Corey G, Corey MS, Callanan P, et al: Ethical considerations in using group techniques. Journal for Specialists in Group Work 7(3):140–148, 1982

Feil WW: Group therapy in a home for the aged. Gerontologist 7:192–195, 1967

Finkel SI: Experiences of a private-practice psychiatrist working with the elderly in the community. International Journal of Mental Health 8(3–4):147–172, 1979–1980

Finkel S: Group therapy: the elderly patient: what helps? Audio-Digest—Psychiatry, 1981

Finkel S, Fillmore W: Experiences with an older group at a private psychiatric hospital. J Geriatr Psychiatry 4:188–199, 1971

Freud S: Sexuality in the aetiology of the neuroses (1898), in The Standard Edition of the Complete Psychological Works of Sigmund Freud, Vol 3. Translated and edited by Strachey J. London, Hogarth Press, 1962, pp 261–285

Gallagher D: Behavioral group therapy with elderly depressives: an experimental study, in Behavioral Group Therapy. Edited by Upper D, Ross S. Champaign, IL, Research Press, 1981, pp 187–224

Gallagher D, Thompson L: Conceptual and clinical issues in the psychotherapy of elderly depressed persons. Paper presented at the annual meeting of the Society for Psychotherapy Research, Toronto, 1982a

Gallagher D, Thompson L: Treatment of major depressive disorders in older adult outpatients with brief psychotherapies. Psychotherapy: Theory, Research, and Practice 4:482–490, 1982b

Goldfarb AI: Preface, in Promoting Mental Health of Older People Through Group Methods. Edited by Klein WH, Le Shan EJ, Furman SS. New York, Mental Health Materials Center, 1966, pp 11–12

Goldfarb AI: Group therapy with the old and the aged, in Group Treatment of Mental Illness. Edited by Kaplan HI, Sadock BJ. New York, Dutton, 1972, pp 113–131

Goodman R: A geriatric group in an acute care psychiatric teaching hospital: pride or prejudice? in Group Psychotherapies for the Elderly. Edited by MacLennan BW, Saul S, Weiner MB. Madison, CT, International Universities Press, 1988, pp 151–164

Grotjahn M: Analytic psychotherapy with the elderly. Psychoanal Rev 42:419–427, 1955

Grotjahn M: Group communication and group therapy with the aged: a promising project, in Aging Into the Twenty-first Century: Middle-Agers Today. Edited by Jarvik LF. New York, Gardner Press, 1978, pp 113–121

Hartford ME: The use of group methods for work with the aged, in Handbook of Mental Health and Aging. Edited by Birren JE, Sloane RB. Englewood Cliffs, NJ, Prentice-Hall, 1980, pp 806–826

Killiffer EH, Bennett R, et al: Handbook of Innovative Programs for the Impaired Elderly. New York, Haworth, 1984

Klein WH, Le Shan EJ, Furman SS: Promoting Mental Health of Older People Through Group Methods. New York, Mental Health Materials Center, 1966

Krasner J: The psychoanalytic treatment of the elder person via group psychotherapy. Acta Psychotherapy 7 1(suppl):205–223, 1959

Krasner J: Treatment of the elder person, in To Enjoy Is to Live. Edited by Fabricant F, Barron J, Krasner J. Chicago, IL, Nelson Hall, 1977, pp 191–204

Lesser J, Lazarus LW, Frankel RA, et al: Reminiscence group therapy with psychotic geriatric inpatients. Gerontologist 21:291–296, 1981

Levine BE, Poston M: A modified group treatment for elderly narcissistic patients. Int J Group Psychother 30:153–167, 1980

Levinson DJ, Darrow CN, Klein EB, et al: Seasons of a Man's Life. New York, Knopf, 1978

Liederman PC, Green R: Geriatric outpatient group therapy. Compr Psychiatry 6:51–60, 1965

Liederman PC, Green R, Liederman VR: Outpatient group therapy with geriatric patients. Geriatrics 22:148–153, 1967

Linden ME: Group psychotherapy with institutionalized senile women: study in gerontologic human relations. Int J Group Psychother 3:150–170, 1953

Linden ME: The significance of dual leadership in gerontologic group psychotherapy. International Journal of Psychotherapy 4:262–273, 1954

Linden ME: Studies in gerontologic human relations, IV: transference in gerontologic group psychotherapy. Int J Group Psychother 5:61–79, 1955

Linden ME: The promise of therapy in the emotional problems of aging. Paper presented at the Fourth Congress of the International Association of Gerontology, Merano, Italy, 1957

Lothstein LM: Psychodynamic group therapy with the active elderly: a preliminary investigation, in Group Psychotherapies for the Elderly. Edited by MacLennan BW, Saul S, Weiner MB. Madison CT, International Universities Press, 1988

Lowy L: Roadblocks in group work practice with older people: a framework for analysis. Gerontologist 7(2):109–113, 1967

MacLennan BW, Saul S, Weiner MB (eds): Group Psychotherapies for the Elderly. Madison, CT, International Universities Press, 1988

Matorin S, Zoubok B: Group psychotherapy with geriatric outpatients: a model for treatment and training, in Group Psychotherapies for the Elderly. Edited by MacLennan BW, Saul S, Weiner MB. Madison, CT, International Universities Press, 1988, pp 107–120

Meerloo JA: Transference and resistance in geriatric psychotherapy. Psychoanal Rev 42:72–82, 1955

Myers WA: Dynamic Therapy of the Older Patient. New York, Jason Aronson, 1984

Parham IA, Priddy JM, McGovern TV, et al: Group psychotherapy with the elderly: problems and prospects. Psychotherapy: Theory, Research, and Practice 19:437–443, 1982

Rechtschaffen A: Psychotherapy with geriatric patients: a review of the literature. J Gerontol 14(B):73–84, 1959

Riley KP, Carr M: Group psychotherapy with older adults: the value of an expressive approach. Psychotherapy 26:366–371, 1989

Rosin AJ: Group discussion: a therapeutic tool in a chronic disease hospital. Geriatrics 30(8):45–48, 1975

Ross M: Recent contributions to gerontologic group psychotherapy. Int J Group Psychother 9:442–450, 1959a

Ross M: A review of some recent group psychotherapy methods for elderly psychiatric patients. Arch Gen Psychiatry 1:578–592, 1959b

Sakauye K: New treatment approaches for the geriatric patient: outpatient group therapy with the elderly. Paper presented at the annual meeting of the Illinois Psychiatric Society, Chicago, IL, November 1979

Schwartz ED, Goodman JI: Group therapy of obesity in elderly diabetics. Geriatrics 7:280–283, 1952

Shere E: Group therapy with the very old, in New Thoughts on Old Age. Edited by Kastenbaum R. New York, Springer, 1964, pp 146–160

Silver A: Group psychotherapy with senile psychotic patients. Geriatrics 5:147–150, 1950

Steuer J, Mintz J, Jarvik L: Geriatric depression: methodological issues in comparing pharmacology with group psychotherapy results. Conference on psychodynamic research prospectives on development, psychopathology, and treatment in later life. Paper presented at National Institute of Mental Health Center Conference on Aging, Washington, DC, 1982

Steuer J, Mintz J, Hammen CL: Cognitive-behavioral and psychodynamic group psychotherapy in treatment of geriatric depression. J Consult Clin Psychol 52(4):180–189, 1984

Tross S, Blum JE: A review of group therapy with the older adult: practice and research, in Group Psychotherapies for the Elderly. Edited by MacLennan BW, Saul S, Weiner MB. Madison, CT, International Universities Press, 1988, pp 3–32

van der Kolk A: Psychotherapy of the elderly: general discussion: the idealizing transference and group psychotherapy with elderly patients. J Geriatr Psychiatry 16:99–102, 1983

Weiner MB, White MT: The third chance: self psychology as an effective group approach for older adults, in Group Psychotherapies for the Elderly. Edited by MacLennan BW, Saul S, Weiner MB. Madison, CT, International Universities Press, 1988, pp 57–66

White MT, Weiner MB: The Theory and Practice of Self Psychology. New York, Brunner/Mazel, 1986

Wolff K: Group psychotherapy with geriatric patients in a psychiatric hospital: six-year study. Group Psychotherapy 14:85–89, 1961

Wolff K: Geriatric Psychiatry. Springfield, IL, Charles C Thomas, 1963

Wolff K: The Emotional Rehabilitation of the Geriatric Patient. Springfield, IL, Charles C Thomas, 1970

Wolk RL, Goldfarb AI: The response to group psychotherapy of aged recent admissions compared with long-term mental hospital patients. Am J Psychiatry 123:10, 1967

Yalom ID: The Theory and Practice of Group Psychotherapy. New York, Basic Books, 1975

Yesavage JA, Karasu TB: Psychotherapy with elderly patients. Am J Psychother 36:41–55, 1983

Yost EB, Corbishly MA: Group therapy, in Depression in the Elderly. Edited by Chaisson-Stewart GM. New York, Wiley, 1985, pp 288–315

Zimberg S: Outpatient geriatric psychiatry in an urban ghetto with non-professional workers. Am J Psychiatry 125:1967–1702, 1969

Chapter Fourteen

IMPACT OF ADULT DEVELOPMENTAL ISSUES ON TREATMENT OF OLDER PATIENTS

Calvin A. Colarusso, M.D.,
and Robert A. Nemiroff, M.D.

In this chapter, we will describe how adult developmental theory and technique have changed both the treatment of older patients with individual psychotherapy in outpatient settings and the treatment of more debilitated individuals in nursing homes and hospitals. There is often a connection between these two types of patients because elderly patients may become debilitated during the course of outpatient psychotherapy. After presentation of the major developmental tasks of late adulthood (ages 60 and beyond), we shall consider the diagnostic process with older patients and then discuss treatment issues.

THE DEVELOPMENTAL TASKS OF LATE ADULTHOOD

Because an understanding of normal development is critical to work with patients at any point in the life cycle, we begin with a survey of the major developmental themes or tasks of late adulthood, based on their initial presentation in *Adult Development: A New Dimension in Psychodynamic Theory and Practice* (Colarusso and Nemiroff 1981).

Maintenance of body integrity. For the healthy individual, the body in old age can still be a source of considerable pleasure and convey a feeling of competence. Older individuals are able to exercise, diet, and maintain the body in such a state that it will allow them to perform many of the physical and mental functions of which they were capable at earlier phases of development. The normal state for the older individual is not one of illness and debilitation, but of physical health.

Reaction to physical infirmity or permanent impairment. Despite a person's best efforts to maintain his or her body in an optimal condition, eventually every individual must face the consequences of occasional or permanent physical infirmity. The healthy older individual faces the developmental task of recognizing that sooner or later his or her body will become impaired in one or more ways. What that person must do is continue to live as full and active a life as possible in the face of the physical impairment.

Attitudes toward personal death. Whereas individuals in young adulthood (ages 20–40) and middle adulthood (ages 40–60) are preoccupied with the developmental issue of accepting the fact that they will eventually die, healthy older individuals have integrated and accepted the idea that death will come to them one day. They have moved on to the related developmental task of late adulthood: concern about the manner in which they will die. In other words, they are concerned about whether they will die in pain, alone, or with dignity in the presence of loved ones.

Integrity versus despair. Erik Erikson (1963) uses the dichotomy of integrity versus despair to describe a major developmental theme in late adulthood. Every older individual must review his or her life, look back over the years, and make a determination about the quality and usefulness of that life for self and others in the community. If that judgment is essentially a positive one, there is a feeling of integrity. If, on the other hand, that individual's life has been a major disappointment, studded with broken relationships or other significant frustrations, the feeling is one of despair. This development task is described by Robert Butler (1963) as the "life review."

Reaction to the death of spouse or friends. As an individual moves into late adulthood, the death of friends or spouse is a common experience. Dealing with death has gradually become a more familiar experience across young and middle adulthood; now in late adulthood, having to face the deaths of friends or spouse is to be expected. In addition to dealing with such acute loss, individuals must be prepared to fill their lives in new ways and with new people in order to continue to find meaning in living.

246

Attitudes toward and preoccupation with the recent and distant past versus the present and future. In late adulthood, most older individuals are preoccupied with the past as they conduct their life reviews, but the healthy ones continue to live in the present and look toward the future, planning not only for their own but also for the futures of their loved ones after they die.

Ability to form new ties. Healthy older individuals deal with losing spouse and friends by establishing new object relationships. These relationships involve not only individuals in the same age group, but also people in earlier phases of life.

Reversal of roles with children and grandchildren. For almost all people, there comes a time at some point in late adulthood when they are no longer able to take care of themselves and must depend to one degree or another upon others. In the ideal situation, that means gradually relinquishing physical care of themselves to children and grandchildren. This developmental task is of considerable importance for the maintenance of physical and psychological health and may cause considerable difficulty for both the elderly persons and their offspring. Many individuals on both sides of the equation are unable to manage this shift, and often that is the substance of therapeutic work with them.

Companionship versus isolation and loneliness. In relation to the ability to form new ties, older individuals must balance the need for companionship with the ability to be comfortably alone. Many older people are content to spend fair amounts of time by themselves due to an inner sense of comfort and continuity provided by memories of loved ones with whom they shared life's most important experiences. Without this inner sense of comfort and continuity, the experience becomes one of isolation and loneliness.

The role of sexual activity. Many in our society have difficulty accepting the idea that elderly people remain sexually interested and capable. In fact, healthy older individuals continue to have active sexual fantasy lives, to masturbate, and to be involved in sexual activity when partners are available. The major impediments to the continuation of sexual activity in old age involve the availability of partners and the attitudes of family members. Because they generally live longer than men, women in particular often have difficulty finding sexual partners in their later years. Even if they are fortunate

247

enough to do so, they may run into marked prejudice on the part of their children against such relationships.

Retirement—use of time, continuation of meaningful activity, work, and play.   The major developmental task for older people is to continue to use their time so that it provides them with a sense of purpose and self-esteem. For some, that may mean continuing to perform meaningful work, sometimes for fewer hours or with less intensity, until they die or are incapacitated. For others, it may mean retirement—turning their efforts to activities that provide pleasure and personal enhancement. Loss of a sense of purpose with regard to the use of time is usually accompanied by other signs of psychopathology.

Financial planning—attitudes toward self-care, surviving family members, society.   In an ideal situation, men and women who began planning for their retirement in young and middle adulthood find themselves in a financially secure situation by late adulthood. The issue for these fortunate individuals becomes a matter of using the money they have accumulated to provide themselves and their loved ones with comfort, security, and enjoyment. Spending money on themselves or planning to pass their resources on to family and society through wills and other legal instruments is the developmental task—one that is often avoided. However, those elderly individuals who could not provide for their own retirement or who failed to do so are confronted with a harsh reality—surviving—while they abide with the realization that they failed to provide adequately for their final years or the next generation.

Case Example
The patient, a 76-year-old architect who was a widower, came for consultation because of difficulties with both short- and long-term memory. Further, he stated, "I feel a general declining of my mental ability, which affects the quality of my life. I have a great deal of difficulty making decisions dealing with the most trivial details of life."

While he readily participated in the diagnostic process, he maintained—with a twinkle in his eye—a skepticism about psychotherapeutic evaluation, wondering about the ambiguity of the process, about all the unscientific questions about feelings, and about what help talking would ever be. Because of his complaints about memory and mental abilities, both neurological consultation and psychological testing were arranged immediately, including the Wechsler Adult Intelligence Scale–Revised I.Q., the Bender Visual Motor Gestalt Test, the Wechsler Memory Scale, and the full Halstead-Reitan Neuropsychological Test Battery. All tests revealed the patient to be functioning without impairment; in fact, in many areas he was functioning above average. Neurological examination was also negative.

It is our practice to review the results of medical and psychological tests with the patient as completely as possible, making sure the patient understands the results and exploring any possible confusion about his or her condition. In this way, we act as "translators" of medical jargon and make sure there is enough time to discuss fully the patient's anxieties about his or her physical condition.

A comprehensive history of the patient's life was taken, including tracing the stages, tasks, and developmental lines. After being reassured about his mental processes, he revealed that he was having an affair with a 41-year-old woman who was suffering from a manic-depressive condition. He was being harassed night and day by this woman, who demanded nearly constant attention, including frequent sex. When frustrated, she would call his house repeatedly and once drove her car onto his front lawn. He had the idea that since he had sex with her, he was now responsible for "treating" her mental condition. The therapist explored this unrealistic demand he was placing on himself and helped him to formulate reasonable limits in the relationship. Soon his woman friend was in the care of a psychiatrist, the relationship ended, and as his anxiety and depression diminished, so did his difficulties with memory and indecisiveness. It seemed as if he had been saying through his physical anxieties, "Stop harassing me. I'm an old man. I'm getting senile. Stop asking me for sex."

He now entered twice-weekly exploratory psychotherapy, in which an incomplete grief reaction was uncovered revolving around the death of his wife. He recognized a physical similarity between his 41-year-old woman friend and his wife when she was in her forties. His punishment at the hands of the manic-depressive woman was for both his unexpressed hostility toward his wife and his guilt over having sex with the girlfriend. He traced a lifetime of guilt and conflict over sex that was related to harsh and moralistic attitudes toward sex on the part of his parents. This was also expressed in the transference, as he had a great deal of difficulty discussing his sexual fantasies and masturbation with the therapist, who he felt sure thought he was an "inappropriate dirty old man." Masturbatory anxiety had again become particularly intense since the death of his wife. Discussing this with his therapist brought considerable relief.

Finally they dealt with his loneliness, and plans were made for him to spend more time with his children and colleagues. He completed treatment, his anxiety diminished, his depression lifted, and his memory difficulties disappeared. As he understood more about his sexual and aggressive conflicts and felt better enough about himself to make more appropriate social contacts, his loneliness decreased.

In light of prevailing biases against treating the older patient experiencing memory difficulties in an exploratory psychotherapy, this man could have received superficial attention and not been able to achieve as much as he did. The therapist's appreciation of adult dynamic and developmental factors was instrumental in bringing about a favorable outcome.

THE DIAGNOSTIC PROCESS

We advocate detailed diagnostic evaluations of older patients to collect relevant data and develop clear understandings of the normal and deviant developmental factors from childhood and adulthood that determine a patient's healthy growth or symptoms (Table 14-1). When tempered with a psychodynamic understanding of the patient's intrapsychic conflicts and detailed knowledge of the patient's physical state and environmental interactions, such developmental constructions allow the clinician to develop a comprehensive diagnosis and formulate an appropriate treatment plan. Detailed evaluations are as important for the treatment of older patients as they are for the treatment of younger ones. It is unfortunate that the practice is often neglected because many clinicians feel that older people usually have organic states that are not amenable to treatment. Many psychologically based symptoms may be overlooked by such an approach.

Diagnostic interviews. Interviews with nonpsychotic adults are usually relatively free flowing, with the content determined by the patient, at least initially. Later the clinician elaborates the chief complaint and the history of the present illness by asking questions to

Table 14-1. Outline of the adult diagnostic evaluation

   I. History
      A. Identifying information
      B. Chief complaint(s)
      C. History of the present illness
      D. Developmental history
      E. Family history
  II. Additional Procedures
      A. Medical evaluation
      B. Psychological testing
 III. Diagnostic Impression
 IV. Treatment Plan
  V. Summary Conference

---

fill in the gaps. The goal is to acquire enough information to understand and describe each symptom, to obtain a chronological picture of its development, and to understand the environmental and intrapsychic factors that influence its course.

Since the purpose is to understand the factors that underlie the symptoms, the diagnostician should immediately begin to identify relevant infantile and adult developmental themes. For older individuals, this means obtaining a detailed account of the course of each symptom across the years and of the individual's childhood experience. Some clinicians fear that the patient will become very repetitive or circumstantial. A further concern is that the clinician will be overwhelmed by the mass of the material. Healthy older people are entirely capable of describing the course of their symptoms in a precise and clear manner. Circumstantiality, obliqueness, or wandering discourse are signs of psychopathology, which the clinician should be able to manage, ensuring that the flow of information from the patient is useful in the diagnostic process.

Developmental history. Detailed developmental histories are taken routinely in evaluations of children but are usually absent in assessments of adults. This practice continues because of the notion that developmental processes play a minor role in the adult and because of the lack, until recently, of diagnostic tools such as adult developmental theory and an adult developmental history outline to assist in the process. The developmental history provides the information about this particular person that allows the diagnostician to understand the meaning of the patient's symptoms and to construct a suitable treatment plan.

Family history. The family history usually consists of a study of relationships during the formative childhood years. Such information should be complemented by the patient's experience with family members into the adult years up to and including the present. Particular attention should be paid to details of interactions with family members around such critical junctures as separations, marriages, births, deaths, etc. Patients in late adulthood will focus on their adult experience with their families if this information is requested. They will also discuss their thoughts and feelings about parents—usually dead by this time—if the therapist is sensitive enough to inquire and willing to listen. It has been our experience that feelings about parents and siblings remain dynamically charged in older individuals and meaningful from a diagnostic standpoint if the therapist sees this material as potentially useful and does not dismiss it.

Underlying this approach to the family history is the idea that the family of childhood and of young and middle adulthood has not vanished from the patient's life. It remains intrapsychically alive and potent, and it can have considerable import for the clinician in understanding the patient's symptoms and treatment course.

Diagnostic and treatment formulations. Once the clinician has obtained sufficient data, he or she can begin formulating a diagnostic impression. We suggest that the diagnostic formulation be divided into three distinct parts: descriptive, dynamic, and developmental.

The descriptive formulation places the patient's symptoms into generally agreed-upon categories such as those in DSM III-R (American Psychiatric Association 1987). Such a formulation is important for communicating with other clinicians. However, it does not convey a meaningful picture of the patient's healthy and deviant development. For that reason, we feel that a dynamic formulation is also imperative. By using the concepts of intrapsychic conflict, a topographical formulation (conscious and unconscious), and structural theory (id, ego, superego), the clinician can provide him- or herself and others with additional frameworks in which to understand the patient's symptoms.

In addition, we suggest that the clinician formulate the diagnosis along developmental lines, tracing major symptoms and conflicts from phase to phase and relating them to major developmental themes and occurrences throughout the life cycle. Such a formulation provides not only a longitudinal understanding of the individual's health and pathology, but also an in-depth picture of that person's unique human experience.

Treatment recommendations are not random. They follow from conclusions reached after thorough diagnostic evaluation. Adult developmental concepts add a new dimension to treatment planning, ensuring greater empathy, flexibility, and latitude. For example, because patients aged 60 and beyond are recognized as still evolving, dynamic, and forward looking, they are potentially suitable for dynamic forms of therapy, including intense introspective psychotherapy and psychoanalysis. Their current problems are understood not only as recapitulations of an ancient past or as preludes to death, but also in terms of current developmental considerations. Because the goal of treatment is to free the individual to pursue the developmental process, comparable importance is given to such environmental issues as financial planning for retirement, relationships with family, and physical health, as well as intrapsychic dynamic factors. Very close attention is paid to the need for supportive psychotherapy, chemotherapy, and other forms of environmental manipulation. The important thing to note is that all these forms of treatment are suitable for some, but not all, individuals in this age group. Work with family members is essential. They can be pivotal in returning the elderly patient to the developmental mainstream if they understand the nature of the problems and are given some direction by the therapist.

Kahana's Classification

Ralph Kahana (1980) has devised a useful categorical approach to the diagnosis and therapy of older patients by dividing them into three groups: the aging, an intermediate group, and the debilitated aging.

Individuals in the first group are experiencing physical changes in appearance, attractiveness, strength, and agility. They have physical illnesses that are manageable rather than critical, and they are dealing with conflicts over the assessment of and balance between ideal aspirations and actual achievements in the areas of personal development, social relationships, community activities, and work. Important areas for investigation are retirement, the awareness of personal time limitation, changes in relationships with the important people in their lives (including loss of some through death), and the eventual approach of the end of their own lives. In other words, these are the normal and neurotic individuals at the upper end of the diagnostic scale who are struggling with the major developmental themes of late adulthood.

The intermediate group consists of patients whose experience in late adulthood goes beyond the normal or the ordinary. They are coping with major changes stemming from physical or mental illness; with the loss of significant individuals in their lives through death, divorce, or other circumstances; and with work or retirement. Some of their significant physical and psychological symptoms are reversible while others are not.

The third group, and the most impaired, are the debilitated aged. According to Kahana, they show the effects of chronic illnesses, diminished functioning of various organ systems, manifestations of brain damage, significant constriction of activities, and an inability to maintain themselves without ongoing assistance from family or community resources.

In reviewing his clinical experience with these groups, Kahana finds depression present in all three. However, the depression becomes more significant and more difficult to treat as one moves from the first group to the third.

We have presented Kahana's typology of patients to illustrate the way in which developmental knowledge and the assessment of organic and psychological issues can be organized as an aid to treatment planning. The first group of individuals is entirely capable of engaging in various forms of insight-oriented psychotherapy or psychoanalysis. The goal is to enhance their developmental process as much as possible by the removal of blocks to ongoing development. For the intermediate group, treatment strategies will range from crisis intervention to forms of insight-oriented psychotherapy. These approaches may be combined in the same individual and used at various times. The psychological clinician must pay particular attention to physical health and illness. Often the clinician must coordinate efforts of the individual and the family to ensure that physical factors are given adequate attention. With the debilitated aged groups, Kahana finds that therapeutic strategies revolve around measures for basic support and for the maintenance of these individuals in as supportive a setting as possible. Considerable work may be done with the individuals who take care of such patients, including their families, in trying to make the patients' lives as rewarding as possible.

Case Example
This is an abbreviated example of the diagnostic evaluation of an 83-year-old man. The problems are extremely common; the diagnostic and treatment considerations equally so. The information was gathered during the 45-minute sessions with Mr. A's children and three individual sessions with the patient.

I. History
A. Identifying Information: The patient was an 83-year-old male whose wife of 63 years had died 6 months before. A retired accountant, Mr. A. lived alone in the house he and his wife had purchased 35 years before. He had two married children, aged 60 and 58, who lived nearby. They had made the initial contact.
B. Chief Complaint: "Dad is forgetful. He isn't eating properly, and he's never gotten over Mom's death. We think he needs help but he doesn't want to come to see you."
C. History of the Present Illness: The patient's symptoms of depression and withdrawal began about 2 years ago, at the time that his wife's health began to decline seriously. The depression (clearly reactive in nature) intensified as she became sicker, and it reached a peak after her death. "I really miss Rose. Taking care of her was hard. I hated seeing her suffer. Now that she's gone I don't know what to do with myself." Weight loss of 40 pounds was more recent, only becoming obvious during the 6 months since his wife's death. "I don't have much of an appetite, but when I do there isn't much worth eating in the house. Rose did all the cooking." In contrast to his children's opinion, Mr. A. did not feel

254

he was forgetful. "I'm not forgetful. I'm just not interested in much these days. I spend a lot of time with my thoughts about Rose and what our life used to be like." Various attempts by Mr. A.'s children to get him to eat and "cheer up" were unsuccessful. They were afraid to leave him alone any longer, but he refused all attempts to get him to move into one of their homes or a nursing home.

D. Developmental History: Each developmental phase, from birth onward, was explored with Mr. A. and his children. Childhood phases, well recognized and understood by most clinicians, will be summarized; relevant adult developmental history will be considered more fully.

Childhood: Mr. A. was an only child, born into an intact family. There was no evidence of significant physical problems at any point in childhood. His mother was involved in his care full time in infancy and early childhood. The patient was not a bed wetter but did recall being told that he sucked his thumb until age 8. He was a good student in elementary school and had many friends. In high school he "played football, dated girls, and studied, in that order." The one traumatic event in childhood, which he recalled vividly, was the sudden death of his mother when he was 8. "It took me a long time to get over that." His father remarried when the patient was 10. He had a "good" relationship with his stepmother, who died 3 years ago.

Young Adulthood (20–40): Mr. A. married his college sweetheart at age 20. After graduation he went to work for a large accounting firm, continuing there for 15 years. At age 35 he started his own business and developed mild depression (untreated) when the business failed. His marriage, "a very good one," was at the center of his emotional life during young and middle adulthood. Mr. A. enjoyed his children, who were born in his 20s, but both he and they described him as a caring but uninvolved father. Mr. A.'s major hobby was golf. He was good at it, and it consumed much of his free time, to the dismay of his wife and children. His children described him as "a physical fitness nut before there were any."

Middle Adulthood (40–60): Both children recalled Mr. A.'s depression at age 55 when their mother developed cancer, which was subsequently cured by surgery. He refused treatment, and the depression lifted spontaneously when his wife recovered. His children described their father's attachment to his wife as total. The couple was very close, almost to the exclusion of their children, now grown, and their friends. Mr. A.'s involvement with his grandchildren was cordial and occasional, not unlike his relationship with his own offspring when they were young. After his business failed, Mr. A. took a job with an accounting firm, remaining there in a middle-management position until he retired at age 65. He described his work as "a job. I made my try for the big bucks and I failed, so I settled for less." His physical health remained excellent throughout his adult years. In fact, he had never been hospitalized in his 83 years.

255

Late Adulthood (60–present): Mr. A. liked retirement and spent his time at home with his wife or playing golf. His interest in friends and family did not increase along with his free time. "I was content to stay at home with Rose," he said. "I never needed much more than that." This pattern continued until his wife's illness and death.

E. Family History: As previously described, Mr. A. was an only child, raised by loving middle-class parents. His mother's death when he was 8 changed his attitude toward life although it apparently did not produce symptoms. After he left home for college, he maintained a distant but cordial relationship with his father, stepmother, and half-brother until his father died when Mr. A. was 45. After that he had even less involvement with his stepmother and half-brother.

II. Additional Procedures

Mr. A. refused both medical evaluation and psychological testing. He was concerned about his weight loss but preferred to eat more rather than be evaluated. He did not plan to begin psychotherapy and saw no reason for testing.

III. Diagnostic Impression

A. Descriptive: DSM-III-R Dysthymia 300.40

B. Dynamic: Mr. A. was deeply traumatized by the sudden death of his mother when he was 8. He used the defense mechanisms of repression and isolation to avoid the mourning process and withdrew from close emotional involvement with others until he met his wife. Her death was much more than a recapitulation of the childhood trauma; it disrupted his most significant object relationship, which had sustained him for 63 years. Deprived of his basic source of security and companionship, he became depressed and regressed.

C. Developmental Diagnosis: Mr. A. got off to an excellent start in life physically and psychologically. Loved and nurtured in infancy and childhood, he developed a solid sense of self and an intact personality. His mother's death during the latency years led to an arrest along the developmental line of separation from infantile objects. From then on, Mr. A maintained a defensive distance from all significant objects in his life—with the exception of his wife—so as not to be hurt again. His development proceeded smoothly along most developmental lines in adolescence, and he was able to get an education, work, marry, and raise a family—but always from a protective distance. This partly adaptive, partly neurotic equilibrium continued until the death of his wife of 63 years.

IV. Treatment Plan

A. Individual psychotherapy for Mr. A.

B. Try to keep Mr. A. in his home as long as he is physically able by providing him with a full-time housekeeper to cook and clean. Encourage his involvement with friends and senior organizations (which he and his wife had attended prior to her illness). Have members of the extended family be in touch on a daily basis, involving him in activities as much as possible, despite his reluctance. Recognize that his need to mourn for his wife will extend for many more months because in late adulthood, particularly if the spousal relationship had existed for many years, mourning takes longer and is not the same process, qualitatively, as in younger people.

    C. If the above fails, consider having him live with either of his children, despite his reluctance.

    D. As a last resort, consider a nursing home.

V. Summary Conferences

    The above recommendations were presented, separately, to Mr. A. and his family. The recommendations for psychotherapy and a full-time housekeeper were eventually but reluctantly accepted by Mr. A. Three months later, he remains in his home, has gained five pounds, and is beginning to trust the therapist enough to discuss some of his feelings about the loss of his wife. The short-term prognosis is fair to good.

ISSUES IN THE TREATMENT OF THE ELDERLY

Transference and Countertransference

Clinicians must have a broad conceptual understanding of transference and countertransference phenomena in order to work effectively with older patients. In discussing these issues we shall focus on two major themes: multigenerational (or reversed) transference and countertransference patterns.

Multigenerational transference. The clinician who works with elderly patients is the object of powerful transference feelings from all stages of the life cycle. Such circumstances require an understanding of sometimes unusual transference phenomena, a considerable degree of empathy, and much personal and therapeutic flexibility.

One of the most common forms of multigenerational transference encountered in elderly people is reverse transference. Instead of reacting to the therapist as a parent figure from the infantile past, the elderly patient treats the younger therapist as his or her child. This transference configuration is based on two major experiences. One is the infantile experience of the patient as child, now reversed in the transference. The other, which often dominates, is the patient's experience as a parent in young, middle, and late adulthood.

A second kind of transference frequently found in the treatment of elderly patients is their tendency to behave as if the therapist were the spouse of many years. This kind of transference too has determinants from the infantile past when the young child wished to be in a spousal relationship with a parent. The new factor in the late adult patient is the experience of having been a spouse, and it may be present whether the real spouse is living or dead.

Hiatt (1971) has ordered multigenerational transferences into three categories: *parental transference*, in which the patient treats the therapist as a parent authority and forms a child-parent relationship with him or her (this is what therapists think of as typical transference, seen in all patients); *peer or sibling transference*, in which the patient puts the therapist in the role of the living or deceased spouse, a confidant, a close colleague, or a younger or older sibling; and *child, child-in-law, or grandchild transference*, commonly seen in older patients, in which the patient manifests a superior attitude toward the therapist, treating him or her as a student, someone to be taught and educated. Such a transference often serves to defend against strongly denied dependency feelings.

Hiatt also finds erotic transference elements to be as common with elderly patients as with younger patients and present in all three forms just described.

Countertransference. All the typical forms of countertransference found in the treatment of younger individuals are present in the treatment of elderly people. In addition, there are forms that relate directly to the older patient's age and position in the life cycle. Therapy is usually conducted by individuals either entering middle age or in middle age, who are themselves dealing with physical changes, significant losses, awareness of time limitation, and personal death. These issues are usually being confronted when the therapist no longer has the benefit of his or her own ongoing analysis to help with countertransference responses.

A major factor in countertransference responses to older patients is the patient's relative nearness to death. This forces the young adult and particularly the middle-aged therapist to deal with the prospect of losing his or her own loved ones and eventually the self to death. In our experience, many therapists entirely avoid the treatment of older patients for this reason.

A second form of countertransference encountered in working with elderly patients relates to their active intrapsychic and actual sexual activities. As do most individuals, the therapist may need to deny the presence of powerful sexual feelings in the elderly patient. This is usually based on unresolved feelings toward the sexuality of one's own parents, stemming from both childhood and adult experience with them. In addition, the middle-aged therapist is undergoing changes in his or her own sexual responsiveness and activity, so the prospect of dealing in detail with the sexual life of the elderly patient may undermine ongoing attempts to establish a new equilibrium in this area.

Hiatt (1971) categorized countertransference reactions as follows:

1. An omnipotent or unrealistic hope—The therapist denies the realistic infirmities of his patient, imputes more strength to the patient than exists, and denies his own fears of death.
2. The feeding of one's narcissism and gaining personal gratification—Some older patients tend to hold their therapists in awe. The therapist must guard against the narcissistic gratifications that come from such a position in the patient's life and not avoid dealing with this aspect of the transference/countertransference paradigm.
3. An unrealistic anger and desire to avoid work with older patients— Older patients are often very difficult and demanding. They may be resistant, regress, or demonstrate overly dependent behavior, all of which can provoke countertransference responses of anger and withdrawal.
4. A feeling of pity and sorrow for a person at the end of life—If the therapist becomes deeply involved with the realistic problems of the patient, he or she may be overly supportive and may attempt to manage the patient's life in ways that preclude helping the patient explore thoughts and feelings about a difficult reality.

Limited Object Ties, Termination, and Death

Elderly patients are often quite limited in the number and quality of their relationships with other people. A spouse may be dead or debilitated. Although attentive, children may be separated by distance or preoccupied with their own lives. Because of such limited object relationships, the therapeutic relationship is often critically important to elderly patients. Positive transference themes may become extremely intense early on and are often difficult to resolve because the patient is reluctant to give up the pleasures that come from the relationship with the therapist. Negative transference may be particularly difficult to analyze, again because of the patient's reluctance to jeopardize a valuable and treasured relationship. The patient may even wish to continue therapy for an unduly long time because it represents the continuation of life itself. Termination involves the realistic loss of a sustaining object tie and may symbolize death.

It is not unusual for a physically healthy patient to become signif-icantly impaired during the course of the treatment. When such a situation occurs, we believe it is incumbent upon the therapist to maintain the therapeutic relationship, altering it to account for the patient's limitations, and to continue to work with the patient, help-ing if necessary with the ultimate developmental task—facing death. The therapist who has formed a significant relationship with the patient may be in a unique position to help that person engage this final developmental challenge with dignity, understanding, and em-pathy.

New Techniques in the Treatment of the Elderly

A number of theorists and clinicians have described techniques that are especially useful in the treatment of elderly patients. We would like to describe several of them.

The first may be called the adaptive value of reminiscence. George Pollock (1981) describes several ways in which reminiscence is im-portant for work with elderly patients. These include communication, self-therapeutic attempts, and adaptation. Pollock writes (p. 280),

> The recollections or fantasies of the past expressed in reminiscences help the elderly maintain a sense of continuity between past and present and between inside and outside. The events, relationships, and feelings re-called also maintain a sense of "me-ness." These recollection-reminis-cences bridge time and maintain the sense of individual personality, especially when there is an inner awareness of diminishing ego intact-ness and competency. In some individuals, the frequently repeated tales of the past are similar to the repetitions, remembering, and working-through sequences observed in the psychoanalytic treatment situation. In some, the obsessive reiteration and recounting is similar to mourning work where recalling-and-expressing is part of the self-healing process. In some elderly, the recounting allows the investigator to observe the consistencies of the accounts as they are restated. . . . I found that rem-iniscence is a way of returning to the past, especially to periods of life when satisfactions and mastering took place. In some, the return is to past traumatic situations where attempts to "work through" these past, but still present, intense mental and emotional disturbances seem clear. The insight of the psychoanalytic observer allows for understanding the meaning of what is otherwise considered "the ramblings of old men and women."

As mentioned earlier, many therapists are hesitant to engage the elderly in reminiscence for fear that the older patient will remain endlessly preoccupied with a boring distant past. In our clinical experience, this is not usually the case. Many elderly individuals will begin the treatment process with a preoccupation with the distant past. However, if they find the therapist willing to follow them in an interested manner, the clinical material may move very quickly into more current areas, thus linking the past with the present in fruitful ways.

The most systematic approach to reminiscence in therapy with older patients has been described by Robert Butler and his co-workers (1963). Butler sees the life review as an important developmental process in late adulthood. Butler and Lewis (1977) define the life review as "a universal mental process brought about by the realization of approaching dissolution and death that marks the lives of all older persons in some manner as their myths of invulnerability or immortality give way and death begins to be viewed as an imminent personal reality" (p. 165).

In our opinion, the life review is one of the major normative developmental tasks of late adulthood. As with any other major process at any point in the life cycle, engagement of the task may lead to developmental progression or developmental arrest. The analysis of the life review often occupies a central place in the treatment process.

Butler and Lewis (1977) describe several techniques for the therapeutic use of the life review. The first involves asking the patient to write or tape various aspects of an autobiography. Conducting the life review in this organized fashion allows the therapist to notice particular areas of emphasis and, equally important, of exclusion.

In addition, Lewis and Butler encourage pilgrimages. In person or through correspondence and photographs, the patient is able to rediscover the personal past and to reconnect with the realistic aspects of that past that still exist. Such steps provide continuity between the present and the past and are often organizing as well as emotionally rewarding. Reunions are particularly helpful pilgrimages in this regard.

Genealogical research provides interesting information about ancestors and a multigenerational link between the patient's life and the lives of those who have gone before. The preservation of ethnic identity is another way to help older patients maintain a sense of continuity and identity.

Scrapbooks, photo albums, and other memorabilia are useful adjuncts to treatment, which can facilitate the therapeutic process when studied together by therapist and patient.

The last area described by Lewis and Butler is a concentration on the individual's life work, a major organizing factor for many with regard to identity and self-esteem during the second half of life.

Techniques for Treatment of the Debilitated Elderly

Goldfarb (1955, 1967) and Goldfarb and Sheps (1954) describe techniques for the treatment of the debilitated elderly. They are speaking of individuals, usually residents of nursing homes, who have suffered somatic, intellectual, or socioeconomic and personal losses. In these individuals they base their psychotherapeutic techniques on the following considerations: 1) Fear and rage have been observed, arising from increased helplessness. 2) Because of this helplessness, the aged sick usually ascribe parental powers to the therapist, identifying him or her with strong figures from the past and present. 3) The behavior of these patients (in response to helplessness) appears to be motivated by a desire to obtain pleasure through mastery by dominating and controlling others.

Goldfarb and Sheps (1954, p. 183) cast the therapist in the role of powerful parent with these increasingly helpless patients in order to help restore and foster self-esteem.

> By utilizing the role that the security-seeking aged sick force on him, guilt, fear, rage and depression can be ameliorated or their social manifestations altered. The patient's sense of helplessness is then decreased. Some successes in performance which follow tend to further increase the patient's sense of worth and strength. Therapy consists of brief (five to fifteen minutes) sessions which are as widely spaced as the status and progress of the patient permits. Each of the interviews is "structured" so that the patient leaves with a sense of triumph, or victory derived from having won an ally or from having dominated the therapist. The therapist attempts to have the patient leave not with the feeling of guilt but of conquest (triumph).

In his contribution to our book *The Race Against Time* (Nemiroff and Colarusso 1985), Gene Cohen describes the psychotherapeutic treatment of an 80-year-old patient. Dr. Cohen followed his patient for several years, both when she was a very active, vibrant woman and after she suffered a major stroke that left her severely demented. We focus here on his ingenuity in working with the patient and staff following her stroke.

Case Example

Mrs. C. had not only lost touch with her personal history, but she had also lost her ability to convey her own history to others. In this regard, we all have a compound history, a two-faceted history—a history of ourselves as we know it and a history of ourselves as others know it. Not to be known by others, to be in effect without a history by being unable to convey one's past, puts a person at a severe disadvantage in eliciting the understanding and empathy of others; a competitive edge has been lost. Here, the therapist can be enormously helpful in conveying the individual's personal and dynamic history, his or her clinical biography. I then attempted to restore some of this competitive edge, this most interesting human phenomenon—Mrs. C.'s history, her biography. Scrapbooks, photos, news clippings, and other personal items of memorabilia were gathered in the process of trying to portray a sense of the patient's past to the staff dynamically. The impact was pronounced. When I returned the next week, there was considerably more verbal and nonverbal engagement between the staff and Mrs. C. And, as more time passed, it became apparent that in addition to the staff's feeling more in touch with the patient because of their knowledge of her personal history, fragments of disjointed thoughts she would express were somewhat better understood due to the enlarged frame of reference in which they were heard.

The problem of imparting Mrs. C.'s history was a much more complicated idea than what has been described. This was because of the dual problem of there being more than one shift of personnel during the course of each day and substantial staff turnover (particularly nursing assistants at nursing homes) during the course of the year. How, then, can one practically convey the patient's history in a dynamic manner described for each shift and for ongoing new staff? Certainly, it is difficult to achieve this effect with a typical chart history; the length involved might preclude many from reading it. It was felt then that one could take advantage of the new technology of audio- and videocassettes and record the history on one or the other of these media. For some institutions there would be the resources to develop a program of audiovisual histories. In other settings, the costs might be prohibitive, but audiocassette histories could still be feasible. Staff at all shifts might be much more likely to obtain these histories due to ease of access—listening to or watching a cassette presentation as opposed to pondering over a chart. Family members could also assume an important role here and probably derive much satisfaction by contributing to the information and presentation on the cassettes. Especially if a given family member is a good storyteller, they should be involved in giving the patient's biography. The experience could be rewarding all the way around. And, in this case example, it might be appreciated that in patients with severe dementia the role of biography can be as important as that of biology in the overall approach to treatment.

The elderly as a whole present mental health practitioners with a wide range of problems and therapeutic considerations (Cohen 1982). In the case of Mrs. C. we see the potential clinical diversity that sometimes can occur with a single older person.

CONCLUSION

In this chapter we have described the major developmental tasks of late adulthood and related them to diagnostic and therapeutic work with patients in this age group. Work with elderly patients is still relatively rare in the mental health professions, pursued by only a few. It is our hope that books like this one will help eliminate the prejudices and provide the theory and clinical techniques that will allow mental health professionals to enjoy working with this rapidly expanding segment of the population.

REFERENCES

American Psychiatric Association: Diagnostic and Statistical Manual of Mental Disorders, 3rd Edition, Revised. Washington, DC, American Psychiatric Association, 1987

Butler RN: The life review: an interpretation of reminiscing in the aged. Psychiatry 26:65–75, 1963

Butler RN, Lewis MI: Aging and Mental Health: Positive Psychosocial Approaches. St. Louis, MO, CV Mosby, 1977

Cohen GD: The older person, the older patient, and the mental health system. Hosp Community Psychiatry 33:101–104, 1982

Colarusso CA, Nemiroff RA: Adult Development: A New Dimension in Psychodynamic Theory and Practice. New York: Plenum, 1981

Erikson EH: Childhood and Society, 2nd Edition. New York, WW Norton, 1963

Goldfarb AL: One aspect of the psychodynamics of the therapeutic situation with aged patients. Psychoanal Rev 42:180–187, 1955

Goldfarb AL: Psychiatry in Geriatrics, Medical Clinics of North America. Philadelphia, PA, WB Saunders, 1967

Goldfarb AL, Sheps J: Psychotherapy of the aged. Psychosom Med 15(3):181–195, 1954

Hiatt H: Dynamic psychotherapy with the aging patient. Am J Psychother 25:591–600, 1971

Kahana RJ: Psychotherapy with the elderly, in Specialized Techniques in Individual Psychotherapy. Edited by Karasu TB, Bellak L. New York, Brunner/Mazel, 1980, pp 305–324

Nemiroff RA, Colarusso CA: The Race Against Time: Psychotherapy and Psychoanalysis in the Second Half of Life. New York, Plenum, 1985

Pollock GH: Reminiscence and insight. Psychoanal Study Child 36:278–287, 1981

Chapter Fifteen

PSYCHOANALYTIC PSYCHOTHERAPY AND PSYCHOANALYSIS WITH OLDER PATIENTS

Wayne A. Myers, M.D.

W hile there were occasional reports in the early analytic literature about psychoanalyses or psychoanalytic psychotherapies
with older patients (Abraham 1919; Grotjahn 1940, 1951, 1955; Meerloo 1953, 1955; Segal 1958), these were infrequent until recent years.
One important reason for the paucity of such case studies was Freud's
specific interdictions (1898, 1904, 1905) against analyzing people over
the age of 50. These interdictions were based on his presumption that
the time period involved in working through the copius amount of
material presented by such patients would be prohibitive. It was also
his belief that older individuals were essentially "ineducable" due to
an "inelasticity" of their mental processes.

In the past decade, an increasing number of reports of analyses and
analytic psychotherapies has appeared (Cath 1984; King 1980; Muslin
1984; Myers 1984, 1985, 1986, 1987, 1988; Nemiroff and Colarusso
1985; Sadavoy and Leszcz 1987; Sandler 1978). The growing body of
published cases is linked to a number of factors. These include the
recognition by dynamically oriented psychotherapists that the defenses in older individuals are frequently more malleable than those
in younger ones. In addition, the realization that older people are
physically healthier and experience a greater life expectancy than
they did in the past has also influenced decisions to embark on long-
term treatments with them. Finally, many such individuals have both
the financial resources and the motivational desire to seek out these
therapies to effect meaningful characterological changes in their
lives.

HOW TO DECIDE WHICH PATIENTS SHOULD HAVE PSYCHOANALYTIC PSYCHOTHERAPY AND PSYCHOANALYSIS

In deciding which individuals should be recommended for psychoanalytic psychotherapy and which should be recommended for psychoanalysis, we frequently find ourselves evaluating patients in terms of a variety of rather inexact and often seemingly confusing concepts. As a result of this, the success in predicting which patients of any age range will do well in either treatment has been quite limited in the past (Appelbaum 1978; Bachrach and Leaff 1978; Bachrach et al. 1985; Erle 1979; Erle and Goldberg 1979; Kernberg et al. 1972; Weber et al. 1985a, 1985b, 1985c). It is obvious that more detailed studies, such as ones correlating DSM-III (American Psychiatric Association 1980) diagnosis and dream frequency data with outcome of treatment (Myers and Solomon 1989a, 1989b), are sorely needed.

Evaluating Object Relationships

Based on the current wisdom in the field, however, probably the most important variable to be evaluated in determining which treatment to recommend involves an assessment of the patient's level of object relatedness. This is best done by taking a detailed history of the individual's lifelong interactions with other people.

For example, Mr. A, a 67-year-old male, presented for treatment with a history of depression in the 2 years following his mandatory retirement from his job. He had been married to his wife for over 40 years, and despite feeling that their sexual relationship had never been a very gratifying one, he did look on her as a person whom he deeply respected. He saw her as a "good friend," someone who was available for him to talk to about emotional issues, if only he were more able to do this.

Prior to his marriage, Mr. A had been involved with only two other women in his life. One relationship took place during his high school years and the other was when he was in college. In both instances, he had felt quite deeply involved with the young women in question, and the relationships had gone on for a number of years. Simply stated, the patient had been an individual who had practiced serial monogamy throughout his lifetime with women to whom he had become deeply attached, despite the limitations on his capacity for intimacy, of which he was aware.

Moving beyond the sphere of his love relationships, Mr. A described having had a number of close and enduring friendships dating back to his college and military service days. These were of great importance to him. He also maintained frequent pleasurable contacts with his siblings, children, and grandchildren. In essence, then, Mr. A was an individual who had demonstrated a lifelong capacity for forming close and enduring relationships with other people. In his description of these interactions, he demonstrated the capacity to recognize and understand the needs and wishes of the other persons involved as being separate and perhaps even antithetical to his own.

If we turn to the case of Mr. B, a 60-year-old man who presented with complaints about his erectile potency with his wife following a case of infectious hepatitis, we can readily see how he differs from Mr. A. Though he, too, had been married for many years, he had never been close to his wife. During the course of the marriage, Mr. B had had many affairs. All of these were short-term sexual liaisons, unaccompanied by any emotional involvement.

In point of fact, Mr. B had actually come for treatment only because of his wife's unhappiness over his inability to perform sexually with her since the hepatitis. Because his wife's considerable wealth enabled him to maintain a lifestyle that he would not otherwise have been able to afford, her unhappiness posed a threat to him. Had his wife not been "on his back," it was clear that the patient would not have come for treatment. To put it another way, he evinced no real sense of caring about his wife's problems. Rather, he was troubled by the possible disruption in his own lifestyle that might result from his wife's difficulties.

Similarly, with his children, siblings, family friends, and colleagues at work, Mr. B felt no real sense of emotional involvement. He perceived people primarily in terms of how they might further his own needs and desires, rather than actually caring about them and their wishes. Though he was an academician, he did not imagine himself as a mentor to his students. Rather, he saw the students, especially the female ones, as being there primarily to gratify his own sexual needs or his desire to be admired.

Hence, Mr. B could be characterized as a narcissistic personality who had thus far not been affected by the passage of time. As such, he can be seen in contrast to those individuals described by Kernberg (1980), who became depressed in middle or later life and consequently become more amenable to treatment by dynamically oriented therapies. During the course of his lifetime, Mr. B had not really felt close to any of the individuals with whom he had been involved. Moreover, he evinced no real conflict about his interactions with others, nor any desire to change himself in this important area of his life. Consequently, we would say that Mr. B's object relationships were rather shallow and need-satisfying and that his potential for benefit in a dynamically oriented treatment was not very good.

Another way to assess a patient's capacity for object relatedness involves an appraisal of his or her interaction with the therapist during the consultative sessions. If the patient expresses curiosity about the therapist's life—for example, if the patient wonders whether the therapist acquired a particular painting or photograph in the office on a trip, or if, in between the first and subsequent sessions, the patient offers a dream whose manifest content seems to contain a reference to the therapist or to the treatment itself—then we may infer that there is some readiness or potential for forming and acknowledging transference feelings toward the therapist. This aptitude on the patient's part is an interactional indicator of his or her capacity to form object relationships. The particular nature of the verbalizations and interactions during the consultative phase may also indicate to us whether the individual being evaluated offers some evidence of a potential for caring and depth in such relationships.

Evaluating Attunement to Unconscious Processes

Another issue of importance in evaluating patients for dynamically oriented treatments is whether they are attuned to their own unconscious processes. Of interest in this regard are specific recollections of dreams and fantasies. Some nascent awareness on the patients' part that such productions may have unconscious meanings, or a recognition by the patients that certain thoughts and actions in their lives are generated by areas of their mind outside the realm of their conscious awareness, is also believed to be a positive indicator of treatability by dynamic methods. Further, perception on the patients' part that events in their lives are influenced by forces within themselves as well as by forces external to them is generally seen as important in determining treatment potential.

Evaluating Depth of Motivation for Change

A further issue of significance in assessing suitability for treatment involves the depth of the motivation for change in the particular individuals evaluated. With many older patients, this is in part determined by the capacity to perceive the time left to them as being finite (Neugarten 1970) rather than infinite, which implies a realistic assessment of the inevitability of their own deaths.

In addition, some perception of the fact that this may be the "last chance" the patient has in his or her lifetime (King 1980) to really change often bespeaks a greater depth of motivation to change and a willingness to withstand the pain and deprivation associated with dynamically oriented therapies. With a number of individuals whom I have seen, some expression of concern over the fact that they are nearing the age at which a parent died and their wish to get more out of their lives than the particular parent did also can be taken as evidence of a desire to change. To state this another way, a person must be painfully dissatisfied with the state of his or her life to warrant embarking upon a long-term treatment geared to changing it.

Evaluating Other Factors

To round out the factors usually taken into account in evaluating the suitability of patients to enter into dynamically oriented therapies, let me note that a reasonable degree of intelligence, some history of success in at least one area of life (such as relationships with others or in work), and a capacity to tolerate strong affects are usually included. Heavy use of drugs and alcohol is generally seen as a contraindication for such treatments.

Clinical Examples of Evaluations for Specific Treatments

If we turn now to just which older patients we should recommend for psychoanalysis and which we should recommend for psychoanalytic psychotherapy, we again find ourselves on uncertain ground. Frequently, there are no clear-cut qualitative differences among the types of patients for whom the different recommendations are made. Rather, we are dealing with quantitative notions when we weigh the ego strengths and resiliency of the individual, his or her age and physical well-being, and the depth of characterological change desired and motivation evident.

All of this leads to specific determinations being made on the basis of the experience and judgment of the individual therapists involved. While this may be acceptable in practice, it is often rather difficult for a therapist to elucidate for other practitioners the specific determinants of his or her choices. In attempting to spell out these determinants, a therapist also quickly becomes aware of the countertransference factors (such as rescue fantasies toward a dead or dying parent) that may actually influence such judgments (Myers 1984, 1986).

Let me turn now to examples of recommendations I have made to older patients regarding psychoanalysis versus psychoanalytic psychotherapy. One such individual, Mr. C, came to see me at the age of 73 because of anxieties over his health. He was suffering from rapidly progressive, severe respiratory disease, with a considerable degree of secondary heart involvement. He quite openly expressed his fears of dying and his anger about the constant struggle for life and breath that his disease had imposed upon him. It seemed unfair to him that he had worked so hard during his life to reach a stage where he could enjoy the fruits of his labor, and now his body had "betrayed" him and consigned him to a limited life expectancy.

While it was clear in taking a detailed history from Mr. C that he had maintained high-level object relationships throughout his lifetime and had gotten a considerable degree of pleasure from his work and sexual life, it was also quite apparent that his major conscious concern during the consultative phase was not related to a desire for profound characterological change. Rather, the dominant theme of his treatment centered on his wish to ward off death. While this desire may frequently be one of the unconscious determinants in an older patient's choice of a younger therapist (Myers 1986), in this instance the wish held center stage.

Though the patient might have been an excellent candidate for psychoanalysis at an earlier time in his life when his health issues were not so overriding a concern, at this stage he was not. The uncertainty of his illness and of his attendant life expectancy, the need for some degree of support from the therapist, and the fact that his primary motivation was for external change rather than for intrapsychic modification led me to recommend a type of analytically oriented psychotherapy for him.

I should note here that I chose a psychodynamic approach because of the need to understand more about the patient's profound anxieties about death. It was apparent to me during the consultative phase that these anxieties were lent an added increment of intensity by factors other than reality ones and that they were causing the patient a profound amount of discomfort. Hence, my recommendation was for an explorative, probing approach rather than for a strictly supportive one.

In the case of Mrs. D, who began to see me at the age of 63 after her second husband left her for a younger woman, my recommendation was different. The patient was a bright, attractive woman, whose underlying physical vigor shone forth despite the surface patina of depression.

Historically, her first husband had died after 10 years of marriage, leaving her at age 31 with two young daughters to raise by herself. Her initial encounter with psychotherapy had occurred at that time and had been helpful in terms of getting her over her feelings of loss

270

and depression about the first husband's death. She did not, however, deal with her feelings of inadequacy vis-à-vis her overpowering mother at that time. The therapy ended when she married her second husband at the age of 33 and had a third child, a son, with him shortly thereafter.

Mrs. D thought of her relationship with her second husband as a rather good one until the time when he left her. The abandonment shocked her out of her fantasy that they would continue to lockstep through life until they died. It also raised the specter of what to do with life now that her children were fully grown and out of the house and she was by herself. In this sense, the lifelong feelings of inadequacy that she had experienced with her mother and with both of her husbands came to the foreground of her awareness, and she felt a tremendous loss of self-esteem. Although she was quite angry with her husband for leaving her, she also felt that she had not measured up sexually during their life together and that she lacked any real substance as a person.

When we examined the nature of her relationships with people, it became clear that she had maintained a number of caring, mutually nurturing relationships with friends since her college days. She had also been a devoted mother and grandmother, and she had furthered her husband's business career by her excellent entertaining and interaction with his colleagues and clients. She also clearly saw her problems as emanating from within herself, and she had ready access to a variety of dreams and fantasies that related to her inner life.

In addition, she wanted desperately to change herself dramatically, so as to be able to get more out of her life and not be as limited as she had been in the past by the feelings of inadequacy. Given this constellation of facts, I chose to recommend that Mrs. D undergo a psychoanalysis with me.

SOME CLINICAL MATERIAL FROM DIFFERENT TREATMENTS

Psychoanalytic Psychotherapy

If we turn back to the case of Mr. C mentioned above, his treatment illustrates a number of interesting features. As noted before, he entered therapy because of his anxieties about dying, which were secondary to his rapidly progressive cardiorespiratory disease. While it was perfectly clear that his life expectancy was realistically quite limited by virtue of his illness, it was also apparent that his anxieties about death did not stem entirely from the current reality factors alone.

A number of ideas that he expressed in the treatment paralleled material described in a paper by Bibring (1966). In that work, Bibring noted that for some individuals, fears of death may involve underlying fantasies of retaliation for aggressive or destructive impulses, the concretization of a masochistic fantasy of total surrender to an overwhelming force or of a claustrophobic fantasy of being covered over or closed in.

In one early treatment session, Mr. C railed on about his fate. This expression of anger was soon followed by a brief silence and then by an overt verbalization of the fantasy that his disease was a punishment for his having been so very aggressive in his business. "I was like the wolf in the three little pigs story," he noted. "I huffed and I puffed and I just blew everyone else away. And now I huff and I puff just so I have enough air to breathe. It's like a case of the punishment fitting the crime."

In this instance, we were able to discover that the genesis of the patient's idea of his illness being a punishment for his aggressiveness had its foundation in his relationship with his father. In one session, when his own associations to the idea of illness as punishment remained enmeshed in present-day realities, I inquired about any prior connections between aggressivity and punishment. He then began to describe some aspects of his early relationship with his father.

"It never occurred to me," he mentioned, "how punitive my father was whenever I stepped out of line and questioned one of his pet ideas or theories. When I left the family business to go out on my own, he couldn't stop predicting doom and gloom for me. He didn't want me to leave him then. I remember how guilty I felt. Only I had to go; I had to be my own man. For months, I used to wake up at night thinking I was being chased by someone or something. Then the dreams went away. Well, he's finally caught up with me now. And this time, there's no escaping the inevitable."

On another occasion, when one of his children suggested to him that it might be more convenient for Mr. C to sell his large house in the suburbs and move into a city apartment, he refused. "I'm going to be closed up in a pine box soon enough," he observed. "No sense rushing things now." When I asked him to expand upon the idea he had just expressed, he revealed a long-standing anxiety about being confined in closed spaces, which antedated the onset of his present illness. He initially related this anxiety to his World War II experiences aboard a submarine being bombarded by depth charges from a Japanese destroyer. We later learned that being confined made Mr.

C feel less "manly" and more "dependent," just as he had felt during a childhood bout of pneumonia, when he first had to be hospitalized and subsequently had to be nursed at home by his mother for a prolonged period of time.

As a result of the elucidation of the aforementioned issues in his treatment, Mr. C was able to feel less anxious about his impending demise. He came to recognize that the intensity of the anxiety his present illness aroused was related to the meshing of the reality factors attendant upon his disease with a number of important themes from his earlier life. In recognizing this, the patient came to feel a greater sense of understanding and control over his life, and he achieved an appreciable easing of his anxiety about his forthcoming death.

In another case, that of Mrs. E, it was also a physical issue that precipitated the dysphoric feelings that led to the referral for psychotherapy. The patient was a 74-year-old diabetic, who suffered from hypertension and advanced diabetic retinopathy. The diminution in her visual acuity made it impossible for her to continue driving her automobile, and she became increasingly dependent on her daughter and her friends to chauffeur her around. In this setting, feelings of depression became quite prominent, and she was referred to me.

After a period of time on antidepressant medication, the acute depressive symptoms were remedied. What remained, however, was Mrs. E's recognition that her life was different from what it had been before her illness. She was no longer the same independent individual she had been before. In addition to not being able to drive alone anymore, she found it hard to pursue her pleasurable hobby of reading, and she could no longer knit things for her grandchildren.

In our treatment sessions, it quickly became clear that the change that was the hardest for her to accept was the enforced dependency on her daughter. "I feel as if our roles have been reversed," Mrs. E commented to me one day, "as if she's the mother and I'm the daughter. It's not as if she's given me a hard time about anything I've asked her to do. Not at all. She's really been a sweetheart with everything. It's more a case of my being the one having the difficulty accepting things."

As she returned to this theme again and again, another dimension became added to the scenario when Mrs. E recognized that her dependency on her daughter smacked of a repetition of her earlier interaction with her own mother. "My mother was also always doing things for me. Even though I'm sure she didn't mean to, I felt like a cripple when I was around her. I don't think I even learned to boil water before I got married. It was terrible."

With this patient, the physical infirmity she suffered in her older age thus reactivated the separation-individuation issues that had plagued her through childhood and on into her young adult life. The agonizing anxiety and guilt that she had originally experienced in going off to college and felt again later when she married were aroused once more in the relationship with her daughter. Part of her desperately wanted the younger woman to be around to help her with essential chores, and part of her experienced the daughter's presence as an infringement on her perception of herself as an adult human being. The resulting conflict was never completely resolved because of the worsening of the patient's physical condition and her enforced dependency on both the daughter and me as her health deteriorated. Her insight into the genesis of her anxieties, however, made them considerably more palatable for her.

Psychoanalysis

If we return to the case of Mr. A described earlier, his enforced retirement at the age of 65 had led to a number of undesirable changes in his life. These modifications in his personality took a couple of years to be noticed by his family, but by the time he was 67 and consulted me for treatment, they were rather well entrenched.

While he had been regarded as something of a lovable curmudgeon when he was gainfully employed, he came to be viewed as an angry downer after his retirement. His waspish tongue, which had been diluted with a considerable amount of humor in the past, was now seen by both family and friends as being quite scathing and not in the least funny. The poisonous barbs he verbalized were most frequently aimed at the considerable job success his two sons had attained.

In his relationship with me, after an initial honeymoon period in which he spoke admiringly about how good my work must make me feel about myself, he began to denigrate me and the practice of analysis. "A helluva racket you've got here, doc," he exclaimed one day. "Getting paid for sitting on your tail and doing and saying nothing. Doesn't strike me as the kind of thing a real man'd want to do."

When I inquired as to his thoughts about impugning my manliness in connection with my work, he initially denied that he had meant anything by his statements. He was only kidding, he observed. Couldn't I even take a joke?

In our session the next day, however, he noted that my calling attention to his comments was similar to what his sons had been saying to him for the past couple of years. Maybe he had meant to knock me down a peg. That was what the boys were always saying about the things he said to them. Maybe he had become more hostile since he had left his job.

After this initial sense of recognition about his own hostile denigration of the masculinity of his sons and of me, he came to see that he himself had felt a considerable loss of manliness in retiring from his job. The aggressive exercise of executive power in his former position had made him feel good about himself and had given him a sense of importance as a man. Without the boost to his self-esteem that his employment offered, and without the presence of any stimulating hobbies or sports to be engaged in during his retirement, he felt unmanned and angry, and he directed his envy and hostility toward the younger men he had the most interaction with—his sons and me.

As the treatment progressed, we came to recognize that issues regarding the patient's sense of himself as a man had been present throughout much of his life but had largely gone unnoticed in his success at work and in his sexual relationship with his wife. Once the work was removed, however, and he began to feel unmanned, his sexual functioning also began to deteriorate, and he felt a considerable decrease in self-esteem.

In his own mind, he came to see himself as passive and dependent, and as looking to others to provide the excitement and aggressivity that he felt was missing within himself. This was reminiscent of his feelings vis-à-vis his father when Mr. A was a child, and it revived his early oedipal struggle with that parent. Needless to say, this struggle with his father was earlier displaced onto his relationship with his sons and then onto me in the transference relationship during the analysis.

As we worked through this issue, he was able to feel better about himself as a man again, and the aggressive envy of his children and of me markedly diminished. When he was finally able to function as a mentor to young men beginning fledgling businesses, he felt he had sufficiently worked through his competitiveness with his father (as displaced onto me and the sons) to contemplate terminating the treatment.

In the case of Mr. F, the patient was nearing his 60th birthday as he presented for treatment. He described a lifelong history of erectile potency, two failed marriages, three prior psychotherapies of little benefit, and a certain shallowness of object relationships, which was worrisome with respect to his capacity to be engaged in a psychoanalytic treatment.

Despite my reservations, a number of positive factors convinced me to recommend a psychoanalytic treatment to him. Among these was the evident warmth he was able to communicate to me in the sessions during the consultative phase. He also revealed a ready attunement to unconscious material, as when he described a dream he had had between the second and third sitting-up sessions. In it, he had the perception that his feet were "mired" (my name being Myers) in quicksand and he was being dragged down into the muck. As he moaned for help, he felt a powerful arm reaching out to pull him free. When I inquired about this, he immediately associated to his expectations from me and the treatment, thereby demonstrating both a potential to form strong transference feelings and the capacity for object relatedness that had not been that readily demonstrable in his past history.

In my further inquiries about this matter, the patient mentioned that his father had died at the age of 60. He attributed the father's early demise to his bottling up his feelings within him all his life, and he spoke of being similar to his father in that regard. He then observed: "If I'm ever going to be happy, now's the time to open up and change things." As noted before, the added amount of intensity given to the motivation to change when certain patients near the age at which a parent died was readily apparent in this instance.

A final factor that influenced my decision to analyze Mr. F had to do with the fact that I unconsciously saw him as a father surrogate at a time when my own father was dying. I did not consciously recognize my wish to rescue him until some months later, when a dream about Mr. F made it quite clear to me. While such countertransference factors may be either positive or negative in working with older patients (Myers 1984, 1986), it is important that therapists working with people in this age range be cognizant of their existence in order not to have them interfere with the treatments.

Again, much of the treatment devolved around the resolution of the patient's tranference feelings toward me. He initially saw me as a young son encouraging him in his quest for masculinity. He wished to borrow my potency to enhance his own. As he then began to succeed more sexually in his relationships with women, I began to be seen as the threatening oedipal father who wished to emasculate him. When this was finally worked through, he was able to achieve a considerable degree of potency with a woman, whom he married and remained happy with until his demise some years later.

The patient's treatment helped me to deal with my own feelings of loss about my father's death. In this regard, I had to deal with strong countertransference feelings for a considerable period of time during the early months of Mr. F's analysis. The most important indicator for me of such feelings was a number of dreams I had about him, which were immensely helpful for me to analyze (Myers 1984, 1986).

CONCLUSIONS

In my own experience and in that of a host of other practitioners mentioned before, dynamically oriented psychotherapies have proven to be of inestimable benefit for many older patients. It is important to be aware of this treatment option in consulting with individuals in this age range, particularly in view of their generally greater sense of physical well-being and their overall greater life expectancy.

To state this another way, it would be a cruel mistake to preclude the consideration of achieving meaningful characterological change in people, simply on the basis of their chronological age. On the contrary, experience has shown that older individuals are frequently more amenable to dynamically oriented treatments than they would have been at younger ages.

In evaluating patients in this age group, criteria such as the degree of object relatedness, of attunement to unconscious factors, and of motivation to change are very important to assess. Some clinical examples of such evaluations and of the resultant treatments have been presented to give a flavor of the tasks involved in treating this group of patients by these techniques.

REFERENCES

Abraham K: The applicability of psycho-analytic treatment to patients at an advanced age (1919), in Selected Papers. New York, Basic Books, 1953, pp 312–317

American Psychiatric Association: Diagnostic and Statistical Manual of Mental Disorders, 3rd Edition. Washington, DC, American Psychiatric Association, 1980

Applebaum S: Psychological mindedness: word, essence, concept. Int J Psychoanal 54:35–46, 1978

Bachrach HM, Leaff LA: "Analyzability": a systematic review of the clinical and quantitative literature. J Am Psychoanal Assoc 26:881–920, 1978

Bachrach HM, Weber JJ, Solomon M: Factors associated with the outcome of psychoanalysis (clinical and methodological considerations): report of the Columbia Psychoanalytic Center Research Project (IV). International Review of Psycho-Analysis 12:379–389, 1985

Bibring GL: Old age: its liabilities and its assets: a psychobiological discourse, in Psychoanalysis, a General Psychology. Edited by Loewenstein R. New York, International Universities Press, 1966, pp 253–271

Cath SH: A psychoanalytic hour: a late-life awakening, in Clinical Approaches to Psychotherapy With the Elderly. Edited by Lazarus LW. Washington, DC, American Psychiatric Press, 1984, pp 1–14

Erle JB: An approach to the study of analyzability and analyses: the course of forty consecutive cases selected for supervised analysis. Psychoanal Q 48:198–228, 1979

Erle JB, Goldberg DA: Problems in the assessment of analyzability. Psychoanal Q 48:48–84, 1979

Freud S: Sexuality in the aetiology of the neuroses (1898), in The Standard Edition of the Complete Psychological Works of Sigmund Freud, Vol III. Translated and edited by Strachey J. London, Hogarth Press, 1962, pp 261–285

Freud S: Freud's psycho-analytic procedure (1904), in The Standard Edition of the Complete Psychological Works of Sigmund Freud, Vol VII. Translated and edited by Strachey J. London, Hogarth Press, 1953, pp 249–254

Freud S: On psycho-therapy (1905), in The Standard Edition of the Complete Psychological Works of Sigmund Freud, Vol VII. Translated and edited by Strachey J. London, Hogarth Press, 1953, pp 257–268

Grotjahn M: Psychoanalytic investigation of a seventy-one year old man with senile dementia. Psychoanal Q 9:80–97, 1940

Grotjahn M: Some analytic observations about the process of aging. Psychoanalysis and the Social Sciences 3:301–312, 1951

Grotjahn M: Analytic psychotherapy with the elderly. Psychoanal Rev 42:419–427, 1955

Kernberg OF: Internal World and External Reality: Object Relations Theory Applied. New York, Jason Aronson, 1980

Kernberg OF, Burstein E, Coyne L, et al: Psychotherapy and psychoanalysis: final report of the Menninger Foundation Psychotherapy Research Project. Bull Menninger Clin 36:3–275, 1972

King P: The life cycle as indicated by the nature of the transference in the psychoanalysis of the middle-aged and the elderly. Int J Psychoanal 61:153–160, 1980

Meerloo JAM: Contribution of psychoanalysis to the problems of the aged, in Psychoanalysis and Social Work. Edited by Heimann M. New York, International Universities Press, 1953, pp 23–35

Meerloo JAM: Transference and resistance in geriatric psychotherapy. Psychoanal Rev 42:72–82, 1955

Muslin HL: Psychoanalysis in the elderly: a self-psychological approach, in Clinical Approaches to Psychotherapy with the Elderly. Edited by Lazarus LW. Washington, DC, American Psychiatric Press, 1984, pp 56–71

Myers WA: Dynamic Theory of the Older Patient. New York, Jason Aronson, 1984

Myers WA: Sexuality in the older individual. J Am Acad Psychoanal 13:88–94, 1985

Myers WA: Transference and countertransference issues in treatments involving older patients and younger therapists. J Geriatr Psychiatry 19:221–239, 1986

Myers WA: Age, rage and the fear of AIDS. J Geriatr Psychiatry 20:127–142, 1987

Myers WA, Solomon M: The frequency of dream presentation in psychoanalysis and in psychoanalytic psychotherapy. J Am Psychoanal Assoc 37:715–725, 1989a

Myers WA, Solomon M: Dream frequency and treatment outcome in psychoanalysis and in psychoanalytic psychotherapy (letter). J Am Psychoanal Assoc 37:1123–1124, 1989b

Nemiroff RA, Colarusso CA (eds): The Race Against Time: Psychotherapy and Psychoanalysis in the Second Half of Life. New York, Plenum, 1985

Neugarten BL: Dynamics of transition of middle age to old age: adaptation and the life cycle. J Geriatr Psychiatry 4:71–87, 1970

Sadavoy J, Leszcz M (eds): Treating the Elderly With Psychotherapy: The Scope for Change in Later Life. Madison, CT, International Universities Press, 1987

Sandler AM: Psychoanalysis in later life: problems in the psychoanalysis of an aging narcissistic patient. J Geriatr Psychiatry 11:5–36, 1978

Segal H: Fear of death: notes on the analysis of an old man. Int J Psychoanal 39:178–181, 1958

Weber JJ, Solomon M, Bachrach HM: Characteristics of psychoanalytic patients: report of the Columbia Psychoanalytic Center Research Project (I). International Review of Psycho-Analysis 12:11–26, 1985a

Weber JJ, Bachrach HM, Solomon M: Factors associated with the outcome of psychoanalysis: report of the Columbia Psychoanalytic Center Research Project (II). International Review of Psycho-Analysis 12:127–141, 1985b

Weber JJ, Bachrach HM, Solomon M: Factors associated with the outcome of psychoanalysis: report of the Columbia Psychoanalytic Center Research Project (III). International Review of Psycho-Analysis 12:251–262, 1985c

INDEX

281